Code Green

A volume in the series
The Culture and Politics of Health Care Work
edited by Suzanne Gordon and Sioban Nelson

Nobody's Home: Candid Reflections of a Nursing Home Aide
by Thomas Edward Gass

Code Green

Money-Driven Hospitals and the Dismantling of Nursing

Dana Beth Weinberg

Foreword by Suzanne Gordon

ILR Press an imprint of

Cornell University Press

Ithaca and London

First published 2003 by Cornell University Press
First printing, Cornell Paperbacks, 2004
Printed in the United States of America

Library of Congress Cataloging-in-Publication Data
Weinberg, Dana Beth.
Code green : money-driven hospitals and the dismantling of nursing / Dana Beth Weinberg ; foreword by Suzanne Gordon.
p. cm.
Includes bibliographical references and index.
ISBN-13: 978-0-8014-3980-3 (cloth : alk. paper)
ISBN-10: 0-8014-3980-9 (cloth : alk. paper)
ISBN-13: 978-0-8014-8919-8 (pbk. : alk. paper)
ISBN-10: 0-8014-8919-9 (pbk. : alk. paper)
1. Nursing—Massachusetts—Boston. 2. Beth Israel Deaconess Hospital Center—Finance. 3. Hospitals—Massachusetts—Boston—Finance. I. Title.
RT5.M4W45 2003
610.73'09744'61—dc21

2003002118

Cornell University Press strives to use environmentally responsible suppliers and materials to the fullest extent possible in the publishing of its books. Such materials include vegetable-based, low-VOC inks and acid-free papers that are recycled, totally chlorine-free, or partly composed of nonwood fibers. For further information, visit our website at www.cornellpress.cornell.edu.

Cloth printing 10 9 8 7 6 5 4 3 2
Paperback printing 10 9 8 7

to my parents, Glenda and Alan Weinberg,

and

to the nurses, for the care they want to give

Contents

Foreword

For almost thirty years, the Beth Israel hospital in Boston served as an icon for the empowerment of nursing. With its chief nurse executive Joyce Clifford working in a unique partnership with CEO physician Mitchell Rabkin, the BI helped to pioneer an innovative model of nursing care called primary nursing, which assigned one nurse to one patient. That nurse was responsible for that one patient throughout a hospital stay and, when possible, during subsequent hospital stays. The hospital also employed an almost all registered nurse staff, hired only RNs with bachelor's degrees, and was committed to enhancing the collaboration between nurses and physicians and giving nurses a greater voice in their institution.

The New England Deaconess hospital, situated just across the street from Beth Israel in the heart of Boston's Longwood Medical area, was also known for a devoted nursing staff that gave excellent care. But it was the BI that shone like a beacon, drawing in nurses from across the globe, who, like weary, sea-battered sailors seeking succor on hospitable shores, yearned for a model of the delivery of nursing services that they could reproduce in their own institutions. For years, the BI served as that model, promising through its strong leadership and committed, satisfied staff to address, and possibly even cure, the many ills that have long made nursing such a difficult and devalued career.

It was thus natural for me to visit the BI and study its best practices when I first started to write about nursing. My first full-length article about nursing, "The Crisis in Caring," written for the *Boston Globe* during the last nursing shortage of the mid 1980s, focused on that hospital. I knew, however, that one article wasn't enough to capture the complexity of nurses' work. When I decided to write a book that followed nurses in their daily work, it was equally natural that I approach Joyce Clifford and ask her if I could follow three of the nurses at the BI for my book *Life Support: Three Nurses on the Front Lines*. Since the BI was one of the only hospitals in which the public relations staff actually promoted the work of nurses, Clifford quickly agreed. I spent nearly three years following three nurses—a nurse in an oncology clinic, a medical clinical nurse specialist, and a geriatric nurse practitioner delivering home care in the BI's home care department—and wrote about the difference that the routine activities of experienced nurses make to patient care.

I chose the BI not only because it had excellent nurses, but also because those nurses received institutional support from the highest levels. What I wanted to show in *Life Support* was that nursing care does not depend on the personal kindness or the moral virtuousness of the nurse. Instead it depends on education and experience and on the institutional support that nurses receive from the hospital in which they are employed. I wanted to show what can happen when nurses receive in-house education, have a voice in hospital policies that affect their work, and have decent—albeit perhaps not optimal—relationships with physicians who treat them like colleagues rather than handmaidens. While the BI had a long way to go in reversing the nineteenth-century template that continues to govern nursing work, it was certainly on the right path. Nurses there were among the most satisfied in the nation, perhaps even in the world.

By the time I was completing my observation at the hospital in 1995, things were beginning to change. Managed care and hospital cost cutting and restructuring had become the trend. In what many believed was a futile and misguided effort to survive in a competitive market dominated by the merger between Boston's two wealthiest and largest hospitals—The Brigham and Women's and The Massachusetts General Hospital—the BI merged with the Deaconess and formed a network with several other hospitals.

Almost immediately nurses began to lose a benefit here, a perk there. Nurses talked about the increasing patient loads and the decreasing managerial and administrative support. Nurses who had been so loyal to their institution that they would never have dreamed of leaving began to quit. Those who stayed constantly complained about the erosion of nursing care in an institution that had once seemed to buck all hospital trends.

As the nurses I knew became more and more despairing, I began to hear another piece of news. In 1999 a young sociologist from Harvard began observing nurses at the BI-Deaconess. She was writing about the fate of the hospital during restructuring and, amazingly, of its nurses, who are often the forgotten players in the new health care drama. She was focusing on what was happening to nursing care. Her name was Dana Beth Weinberg. When she finished, her report began circulating among the nursing staff. Everyone I knew was talking about it. I wanted to see it.

A friend gave me a copy, and I read it with fascination. Weinberg's study, I thought, was far too important to languish on the shelf of a university library where it would be read by the odd nurse researcher or sociologist. It had to be a book—a book widely read not just by nurses but by doctors, policy makers, politicians, health care journalists, and other academics who are interested in the sociology and the organization of work as well as the advancement of women. Thankfully, Dana Weinberg and Cornell University Press have produced that book.

Although *Code Green* is a study of the impact of hospital cost cutting and restructuring on the nursing work provided at a merged hospital, this book is not about one institution. Instead, it uses the microcosm of profit-driven restructuring at the Beth Israel-Deaconess Medical Center to call attention to the larger phenomenon of the cost cutting that has threatened nursing and patient care not only in the United States but across the globe.

A careful reading of *Code Green* demonstrates that the potentially catastrophic global nursing shortage we now face was hardly an inevitable result of an aging nursing workforce or changes in women's roles. It is an artificial creation that was a response to health care cost cutting during the managed care era. Health care consultants eager to take advantage of the fears of hospital administrators—who had become extremely concerned about the level of insurance reimbursement—presented administrators with plans that were supposed to deliver better care for less money. CEOs, nursing executives, and hospital boards of trustees did not adequately question their approach. To illustrate this global trend, Weinberg could not have chosen a better example than the Beth Israel-Deaconess. The fact that a hospital with such strong nursing leadership, such a robust partnership between a chief nurse and a chief doctor, such an educated and satisfied RN workforce, and such an international reputation could become such an easy victim of restructuring and cost cutting should serve as a lesson to all those concerned about providing high-quality patient care.

Weinberg's ultimate message is that the kind of strong top-down leadership so often touted by some nurses as the solution to nursing and its discontents is simply not enough. Leadership is, of course, crucial. But just as nurses' ability to deliver safe patient care is dependent on institutional support, so too nursing leaders' ability to deliver safe and effective leadership is dependent on forces outside the hospital. To be effective, nursing leadership must be bolstered by strong state and government regulations of the hospital industry and by the mobilization of bedside nurses.

Today, as we face the contemporary nursing crisis, nurses are once again discussing the importance of nursing leadership. In the recent report *Health Care at the Crossroads: Strategies for Addressing the Evolving Nursing Crisis* it is clear that the Joint Commission on the Accreditation of Healthcare Organizations rejects government regulation of the industry and promotes instead voluntary solutions to the crisis. As commission members and the public ponder the wisdom of this approach, *Code Green* should be required reading.

The Beth Israel was the prime example of a self-regulated hospital. All its great innovations and models were voluntary creations. While these innovations thrived during an era of more plentiful healthcare financing, they were blown away like straws in the wind with the advent of cost cutting.

The Deaconess was also an exercise in voluntary management. It anticipated and, indeed, paved the way for restructuring by initiating a reengineering effort intended to provide top-notch nursing care that was both less expensive and more efficient. The Deaconess model also collapsed under the weight of profit-driven restructuring. Perhaps Weinberg's most powerful message is that no matter what the care delivery model, when profit and institutional survival are the motives that guide administrative action and behavior, nursing suffers.

In *Code Green,* Weinberg raises questions that should be the subject of reflection and action for many different actors—or stakeholders, in the new market jargon—on the health care stage.

Doctors concerned with the provision of safe care to their patients should read this book and ask themselves why they do not fight harder for nursing care. At the Beth Israel-Deaconess Medical Center, as Weinberg shows, some doctors were so busy fighting with one another that they didn't notice when the patient was lying frightened, alone, and unattended because nursing was systematically disorganized and nurses had become so overwhelmed and demoralized. What is so interesting about this story is that nurses, in fact, served as canaries in the mine for physicians. While nursing care was being dismantled, doctors were also complaining about the eroding conditions of their work. Nurse leaders should also read this book and reflect. Nursing puts great emphasis on the development of administrators who are nurses and nursing leadership. But in an era of cost cutting is leadership enough? During a serious crisis, are managers who once practiced nursing too compromised by their dual allegiance to the hospital and to the nursing staff to provide effective leadership involving issues of greatest concern to working nurses? Similarly, hospital administrators and boards of directors must take responsibility for their actions. Today many administrators and trustees are blaming consultants for the failed policies of the mid-1990s. But consultants didn't magically appear unbidden on hospital doorsteps. As Weinberg shows, with the assent of their boards, hospitals like the BI-Deaconess paid millions to invite consultants into their institutions because they wanted to cut costs. When nurses, doctors, and patients complained that hospitals were cutting care, executives conveniently sidestepped accountability by arguing that "the consultants made us do it." *Code Green* sends a message to these stakeholders—one that they should take very seriously indeed.

Finally, working nurses must also pose serious questions about models of professionalization that seem to be inadequate to deal with the brutal economic realities of today's health care marketplace. The Beth Israel experiment was truly extraordinary and worthy of widespread emulation. But Beth Israel and Deaconess nurses were loathe to join the unions that could have better protected their own professional interests as well as those of their patients. They were suspicious of the kind of protests other more assertive nurses in Boston and elsewhere mounted to alert the public to the dangers of health care cost cutting and profit-driven hospital restructuring. Many BI-Deaconess RNs argued that nurses who were publicizing the dimensions of the nursing crisis to the public were angry and unprofessional. Nurses who read Weinberg's book need to ask themselves whether nursing's emphasis on individual patient advocacy is sufficient to protect patients as well as the profession. In using the title *Code Green,* Weinberg both invents a term and borrows one that is sometimes used in hospitals. By calling a "Code Green" she warns us of the dangers of a market-driven health care system that puts profits over patient care. The term is even more apt because it is used by certain hospitals to signal a facility failure that must be immediately addressed. Now, as the United States fights terrorism, the term is also one of a series of color-coded alerts and warns of the potential for mass casualties.

As studies document, facility failures and the potential of mass casualties are precisely what we are suffering from and will continue to experience if the nursing crisis is not remedied by serious, systematic efforts to regulate the hospital industry so that nursing can finally become a long-term, satisfying career. If, as the Beth Israel model proved, primary nursing, decent patient loads, and a strong institutional voice for bedside nurses are keys to better care for patients, then that model cannot be voluntary. It is a must.

So is reading this book and acting on its urgent message.

Suzanne Gordon

Acknowledgments

I have incurred many debts of gratitude in the course of writing this book. I would like to acknowledge those individuals who played an important role in enabling this study.

Mary-Jo DelVecchio Good generated the initial idea for this research after a short stint in the hospital. She encouraged me to go to Beth Israel Deaconess Medical Center (BIDMC) in Boston to find out, "Why are the nurses crying?" The original project would have been impossible without her support and her belief in the importance and relevance of this research subject. Barbara Reskin, Benjamin C. Amick III, and Jody Hoffer Gittell also provided critical guidance, support, and advice. Their questions, insights, and mentoring shaped this project in more ways than they realize. I am grateful for the attention and commitment that these talented individuals devoted to the improvement of my research and to my development.

A number of individuals at BIDMC enabled this research. Susan Chamberlain Williams, Joyce Clifford, and Trish Gibbons helped me negotiate the internal organization, gain access to key personnel and information, and present my results within the hospital. Susan Chamberlain Williams also met with me regularly to discuss my findings and commented on early drafts. Mary Williams and Jo O'Driscoll assisted me in submitting my study for review to the hospital's review committees and provided ongoing assistance as I modified protocols and procedures related to the survey.

The nurse managers on the six units I studied facilitated my access to staff on their units. They deserve full credit for the success of the focus groups and surveys that I conducted as part of this research. I am grateful to the many individuals who took time from their busy schedules to furnish me with the hospital data I needed. Finally, I thank all of the hospital employees who participated in this research by allowing me to shadow them, participating in focus groups and interviews, and completing surveys. I hope I have done justice to their perspectives and insights.

A number of other individuals also had a hand in promoting my research efforts. With BIDMC's permission, Linda Aiken and Julie Sochalski of the University of Pennsylvania generously shared survey data collected from nurses at BIDMC as part of other studies. They also provided feedback on my initial research design.

A Graduate Research Fellowship from the Sociology Division and a Grant for Doctoral Dissertation Improvement from the Division of Decision, Risk, and Management Science, both from the National Science Foundation, as well as an Eliot Fellowship for Dissertation Completion from Harvard University provided financial support for the original project.

It is an enormous undertaking to turn dry academic research into a book. I thank Fran Benson, Editor-in-Chief at Cornell University Press, for believing that I could do it and being patient, encouraging, and supportive when life events threatened the endeavor. I thank the reviewers for their feedback on an earlier draft. I owe a world of thanks to Suzanne Gordon for her brilliant editorial assistance, her enthusiasm about the project, and her practical advice—all of which helped enliven my prose and bring the manuscript to life. Not least of all, I thank her for generating the title for the book.

I am grateful for the many friends who commiserated and rejoiced with me during the ups and downs of this process. Most of all, I am grateful to my family: my parents, Alan and Glenda Weinberg, my husband, Eugene Shuster, and my daughter Michaela Shuster. Their unconditional love and support sustained me in my efforts and continually reminded me of the value of my achievement.

Code Green

Introduction

In 1998 my then graduate studies adviser, Mary-Jo DelVecchio Good, was hospitalized at Beth Israel Deaconess Medical Center with a life-threatening condition. Soon after she was transferred from the intensive care unit, Good, always the social scientist, could not help but notice that her nurses seemed frustrated and harried. Driven by curiosity and concern even in her weakened state, she began to ask questions and to interview her nurses from her hospital bed. Over the course of her few-day stay at the hospital, she listened to her nurses' stories about their work. Several lamented, "This isn't what I went into nursing for. It shouldn't be this way." They bemoaned that they could not give patients the care they wanted and had been trained to give. Prompted by Good's compassionate listening, these nurses literally cried to her in her hospital room. They sought care and comfort from her even while she needed care and comfort.

For Good, the patient, hearing the nurses' stories must have been a frightening experience. With her body physically weakened by illness, she depended on these crying nurses. She relied on their competence to monitor and evaluate her condition, to recognize signs of relapse, and to make sure she was out of danger. She needed them to bring her the right medications in the proper dosage at the appropriate interval, and she wanted them to talk with her about her condition and what would happen after discharge.

But Good, the social scientist who had spent two decades researching how doctors learn, define, and argue about competence, found the nurses' experience intriguing. On this unit, in this hospital, the nurses found it difficult to do what they as nurses felt they should be doing. Their stories called into question not their own competence as nurses but the competence of their institution to deliver proper care for patients.

Barely recovered from her illness, Good returned to Harvard University with a gleam in her eye. She had sniffed out an important story that needed a writer, and I was a graduate student who needed a dissertation—a perfect match. Good sent me out to discover, "Why are the nurses crying?"

How could it have happened that nurses found their desire and efforts to care for patients impeded by circumstances at, of all places, Boston's Beth Israel Hospital? This, after all, was no ordinary hospital. Beth Israel was not only a Harvard teaching hospital but also one of the finest academic medical centers in Boston. It was the first hospital in the country to establish a patient's bill of rights. And historically it had been one of the best hospitals in the world to be a nurse. At a time when many hospitals treated nurses as a cheap, disposable labor force, Beth Israel refused to do so. It treated nurses not as doctors' handmaidens but as professionals with crucial knowledge and skills to contribute to patient care. It was an exemplar of professional nursing practice, and nursing leaders and students from around the world came to Beth Israel to "see how it's done." In the nursing shortage of the 1980s, the hospital had no trouble filling vacancies. A generation of researchers studied the features of Beth Israel's nursing program and those of similar hospitals, institutions that became known as "magnet" hospitals for their ability to attract and retain nurses (Aiken, Smith, and Lake 1994; Kramer and Schmalenberg 1988). Even among these exemplary institutions, Beth Israel was the prototype, the gold standard. By most accounts, this hospital had been a paragon of competence.

But times had changed. In 1996, just two years before Good's hospitalization, Beth Israel Hospital had merged with its neighbor, the New England Deaconess Hospital. With merger problems and falling reimbursements, the hospital found itself in the middle of a crisis, a state of emergency that I call "Code Green." BIDMC was losing more than one million dollars each week. In response, the hospital scrambled to restructure by streamlining its operations and reorganizing departments. BIDMC was not alone in its desperate need to restructure, nor were the hospital's nurses alone in their frustration with the results.

Across the country, a market characterized by increasing managed care penetration, competition, and restriction of Medicare and Medicaid payments provided the impetus for vast restructuring of health care organizations, especially hospitals, in the 1990s (Barro and Cutler 1997; Kuttner 1999; Robinson 1994; Shortell et al. 1997; Shortell, Gillies, and Devers 1995; Sochalski, Aiken, and Fagin 1997). Over the past decade, American hospitals eagerly borrowed various restructuring strategies from the corporate sector (Fennell and Alexander 1993; Lee and Alexander 1999; Mick 1990; Topping and Hernandez 1991). With shrinking or even disappearing profit margins, many hospitals found themselves in a Code Green. They focused attention on the financial aspects of their operations and sought ways to increase revenues while decreasing costs.

Increasingly, the professional health care workforce began to complain about their hospitals' responses to Code Green. The profit-maximizing behavior of healthcare organizations, they claimed, curtailed their decision-making autonomy and interfered with their ability to provide high-quality care to patients (see, e.g., the national surveys by Donelan et al. 1997; Shindul-Rothschild, Berry, and Long-Middleton 1996). In response to Code Green, hospitals adopted the values of corporate rationality, which entail an emphasis on productivity, cost-effectiveness, and efficiency. In adopting restructuring strategies from industry, consultants and others have guided hospitals to focus on quantitative improvements, emphasizing progress along measurable dimensions in financial and patient outcomes. With corporate bodies and caregivers all using standards and benchmarks to define quality, "care tends to get standardized and restricted to what fits in the boxes of printed forms" (Stone 1999:63; see also Gray 1991). This emphasis on standardization and throughput in health care organizations encourages an "assembly line" form of practice that interferes with the development of provider-patient relationships (Norrish and Rundall 2001; Scott et al. 1995). These conditions constrain providers' ability to respond to their patients' unique situations and needs.

In December 1997, 2,300 physicians and nurses published a call to action in the *Journal of the American Medical Association*. The dire language with which they described the threats of "market medicine" signaled the assault on professional culture brought by increased administrative cost control:

> Mounting shadows darken our calling and threaten to transform healing from a covenant into a business contract. Cannons of commerce are displacing dictates of healing, trampling our professions' most sacred values. Market medicine treats patients as profit centers. The time we are allowed to spend with the sick shrinks under the pressure to increase throughput, as though we were dealing with industrial commodities rather than afflicted human beings in need of compassion and caring (Ad Hoc Committee to Defend Health Care 1997:1733; for related discussion see Good [1995] 1998:xi).

At the heart of this indictment is a protest against the constraints a profit-driven system places on health care providers' ability to choose and to perform the care that they deem is in their patients' best interest. When hospitals adopt the values of corporate rationality, the balance of power in these institutions shifts in favor of administrators and away from care providers (Leicht, Fennell, and Witkowski 1995). For many clinicians, administrative cost control represents an assault on caring and professional autonomy. The divergence in values pits administrators seeking to protect the future viability of their institutions in the midst of a Code Green against health care professionals seeking to provide the care they want to give. The Beth Israel case sheds light on these conflicts. It shows what happens to people who provide care and to those who depend on that care—something often overlooked in restructuring—and provides insight into the current nursing shortage.

In 1996, Beth Israel Hospital merged with its neighbor, the New England Deaconess Hospital, another Harvard teaching hospital, to form the Beth Israel Deaconess Medical Center (BIDMC). At the same time, the two Boston hospitals and Mount Auburn Hospital in Cambridge formed CareGroup, a health care system that would treat one out of every nine patients in Massachusetts.[1] The merger was considered a necessary step to

[1] Peter J. Howe, "Hospitals Complete Deal to Form System: CareGroup Not Planning to Lay Off Any Workers," *Boston Globe,* 2 Oct. 1996, E2, city edition.

compete in the Massachusetts health care market, which was dominated by Partners HealthCare, Boston's first major health care network.[2]

The New England Deaconess and Beth Israel Hospitals hoped to cut costs by integrating the two facilities. They planned to merge the hospital boards as well as all clinical and administrative functions.[3] Public statements by the CEOs of the two premerger hospitals stressed the goodness of the match: both were teaching hospitals affiliated with Harvard Medical School, both placed a premium on quality patient care, and both enjoyed outstanding reputations as institutions providing high-quality care. The initial optimism glossed over profound differences in organizational arrangements around nursing at the two institutions.

Prior to the merger, the New England Deaconess Hospital built a reputation as a pioneer in the general restructuring of hospital care. The small surgical specialty hospital stood on the forefront of streamlining operations and implementing total quality management efforts. The hospital boasted that it increased efficiency and productivity while maintaining care quality and patient satisfaction. One strategy that the hospital used involved cutting registered nurse positions and replacing registered nurses with aides, who took on nurses' more "mundane" tasks (e.g., checking vital signs, bathing patients, and changing bedpans).

The Deaconess's cost-reducing strategy was in stark contrast to the premium that Beth Israel placed on its nurses. Beth Israel Hospital built its reputation around the individualized care that its highly skilled and educated nurses delivered directly to patients. In the 1970s, Beth Israel implemented a practice known as *primary nursing,* in which each nurse became responsible for the care of particular patients from admission to discharge. Even though other registered nurses cared for the nurse's patients during her off shifts, the primary nurse had twenty-four hour accountability for her patients' care. By following the patient's progress through the whole of the patient's stay, the nurse got to know the patient, to recognize changes in the patient's condition, and to plan the patient's care, thereby ensuring coordination and continuity of care. This system emphasized the knowledge and insights that a nurse, through prolonged

[2] Alex Pham, "Mt. Auburn Set to Merge With Hospitals; Union Would Form $1b Health Care Network," *Boston Globe,* 12 Mar. 1996.

[3] Ibid.

interaction with her patients, could bring to bear on their treatment. In line with the value that the hospital placed on nurses' professional knowledge and experience, Beth Israel departed from the practices of many other hospitals. It paid its nurses salaries rather than hourly wages and offered them the opportunity for promotion without having to leave direct service. This was in contrast to most hospitals where a nurse seeking to advance had only a few options—to leave the bedside and become a manager or to go into a career in academia or consulting. Beth Israel implemented a program of clinical advancement: Nurses who expanded their skills and education could climb up four levels of clinical nursing, each of which brought increased pay and respect. (See Gordon 1997 for a full description of primary nursing practice and its historical importance.) Before the merger, one of Beth Israel's ad campaigns referred to the high quality of patient care with the slogan, "It's the nurses." The catchy sound bite largely reflected the culture of clinical practice at Beth Israel. After the merger, however, references to the power of nursing in BIDMC ad campaigns were notable for their absence.

A 1997 *Wall Street Journal* article described the threat that Beth Israel's unique and important nursing model faced from the merger and cost cutting:

> But [the primary nursing] tradition may be in jeopardy. A year ago, in an attempt to boost efficiency and compete better with its rivals in an era of tight medical budgets, Beth Israel Medical Center started merging with Boston's busy Deaconess Hospital. The impact of the merger and other cost-cutting measures, many doctors and nurses fear, could make the commitment to primary nursing too difficult to maintain. And if the concept can't survive at its very birthplace, they say, it may be doomed at other hospitals, too.[4]

The article paints an unappealing picture of what care might look like if the hospital could not maintain its commitment to primary nursing. It contrasts the premier Beth Israel primary nursing practice with the care

[4] Laura Johannes, "On the Ward: Primary Nursing—A Model for Hospitals Around the Country—May Not Be Able to Survive the Push for Efficiency," 23 Oct. 1997, eastern edition R12.

provided at the Deaconess: "Over at the Deaconess side of the hospital, two 'patient-care techs' with three months' training circle the cardiac ward checking patients' vital signs. About a year and a half ago, the Beth Israel side added a nursing student to do some minor tasks . . . but at Beth Israel, for now at least, taking vital signs remains a nurse's duty." The article continues, "In addition to being slightly busier, Deaconess—where a typical nurse with four or five years' experience might make . . . roughly the starting salary at Beth Israel—appears to put less emphasis on nurses' clinical judgments." The key difference between primary nursing and this other model of care is whether patients have the benefit of a qualified nurses' ongoing personal attention and clinical judgment.

Bolstered by the research about the benefits of the primary nursing model for patients and the lavish praise they received, Beth Israel nurses were convinced of the superiority of their model. But critics, particularly from the Deaconess's Nursing Department, faulted Beth Israel's primary nursing practice for being too resource-intensive and, thus, too expensive in the current financial crunch. The merged hospital's worsening financial situation threatened the primary nursing practice Beth Israel Hospital had built since the 1970s.

Events in March 1999 brought the hospital's dire financial situation center stage. Due to merger problems and decreased Medicare payments—a result of the 1997 Balanced Budget Act—BIDMC faced an operating loss of $73 million for the 1999 fiscal year. A team of consultants, working with management to engineer a turnaround plan for the hospital, had been buzzing around the hospital for months. At a Medical Staff Meeting in early March, the hospital leadership finally unveiled the outlines of this plan, which it dubbed "Genesis."

Doctors and nurses filled a large auditorium to listen to a highly produced show given by the BIDMC management team. Angry whispers and murmurs rushed through the crowd as the PowerPoint slides flashed across the large screen. The slides presented detailed plans that many on the medical staff involved in hospital committees had already been suggesting or even working on, such as greater consolidation of the two hospitals. A dark joke circulating after the meeting suggested the widely held perception that the remainder of the Genesis team's plan consisted of nothing more than cutting staff:

Q: What comes after Genesis?
A: Exodus and Numbers. (Fieldnotes, March 1999)

Although there was no reduction in the number of bedside nurses, frontline nurses felt the full force of the Genesis Project's budget reductions over the next few months. Over the next six months, changes at the hospital put the squeeze on frontline nurses by pulling them away from the bedside to perform other duties, increasing their patient loads, and leaving them shorthanded.

An angry nurse questioned the hospital's financial priorities: "It seems to me if we've got a couple of million dollars to spend on the Genesis Report, to tell them what they already knew, that they could have spent that money on patient care." She accused the administration of "backing off from a commitment to good nursing practice" and "playing the actuarial odds" with patients' well-being and "hoping there are not a lot of complications" (July 1999). Another nurse made a similar observation, linking quality-of-care issues to the hospital's current financial focus: "I used to believe that this hospital took excellent care of every patient, and I don't feel like that any more. . . . I think that it's done with the primary focus on being expedient and cost-effective and [getting] patients in and out as quickly as you can because every minute they're here it costs the hospital money to care for them, one way or another." She emphasized that the result was "patched together and shoddy care" (June 1999).[5]

BIDMC management viewed as suspect nurses' claims about threats to patient care. The hospital administration characterized nurses' concerns about quality as mere resistance to change. They diminished the significance of nurses' response by attributing it to a "normal" and "expected" resistance to change. Nothing to really worry about. With nursing at the center of patient care, the old Beth Israel Hospital had structured admission procedures and support services around the nurses' needs in caring for patients. However, BIDMC's financial crisis necessitated an emphasis

[5] All quotations are from the interviews I conducted at BIDMC unless otherwise noted. I refer to all of the nurses and nurse administrators in this study using feminine pronouns because the vast majority of nurses in this study, as in the nursing field, are women. Given the small number of male nurses working at BIDMC, revealing the gender of the nurses in particular quotations might have compromised the confidentiality of the interviews. I have randomly assigned genders to the nonnurse administrators.

on cost-cutting and streamlining measures, such as shortening the length of stay and reducing support services. Administrators recognized that Beth Israel nurses, whose practice had been built around their relationships with their patients, mourned not having the same quality or quantity of time to spend with those in their care. In interviews, hospital administrators offered what became a familiar refrain, "Nurses need to adjust their standards. We can't go back to the way we did things before."

During an interview, I asked a nurse about management's assertion that nurses' concerns about not having enough time with patients reflected little more than resistance to change. She roared at me,

> That's a crock of shit. Change what? Change from giving good quality care to giving no care . . . The things that aren't being done aren't things that you can catch up on later. . . . If you don't see a patient for three hours, you can't somehow later on make up for the fact that for three hours you haven't evaluated the patient. So then you're shooting craps again. They're hoping there's not a complication in that three-hour period where they've got no nursing care. And that has nothing to do with change. That's poor nursing care. And it's poor nursing care that the nurse has no control over because she can't be two places at once.

Her angry response captured the perspective of many of the nurses I interviewed. Although nurses did indeed mourn the loss of the personal relationships that they were once able to develop with patients, their complaints about not having enough time related to pressing concerns in providing patient care. Not having enough time with patients meant not having enough time to evaluate them, to monitor their condition, to understand and plan for their needs after discharge, or to provide basic physical care. For nurses, spending time with patients was not an optional luxury. This was not about the nicety of holding someone's hand or making small talk about their children, but about not being able to provide what they considered necessary care to diseased, weak, vulnerable, and potentially unstable patients.

What happened over the course of three years at BIDMC shows us in microcosm what has happened in our health care system as hospitals have increased the demands on registered nurses while decreasing their time with patients.

From 1981 to 1993, the number of nursing caregivers at the bedside in hospitals declined by 7.3 percent (controlling for the type and severity of patients' illnesses and the rise in volume of patients), even as all other categories of hospital staff increased. Reductions in nursing staff—registered nurses (RNs), licensed practical nurses (LPNs), and nurses' aides—were more severe in states with high managed care penetration: The overall proportion of nursing personnel relative to inpatient volume and severity fell 27 percent in Massachusetts, 25 percent in New York, and 20 percent in California between 1981 and 1993. As a result, nursing personnel dropped from 45 percent of the hospital labor force in 1981 to 37 percent of the hospital labor force in 1993 (Aiken, Sochalski, and Anderson 1996).

In the late 1990s, hospitals began to change the composition of their already reduced nursing staffs by replacing RNs and LPNs with less-skilled nursing personnel, who also command lower salaries (Buerhaus and Staiger 1999). In theory nurses' aides carry out the "mundane" tasks involved in patient care, like emptying bedpans or changing sheets, and free up highly skilled RNs for the more "complicated" tasks requiring their expert knowledge and skills. In practice, however, nurses' aides were assigned the time at the bedside that RNs, while performing so-called mundane tasks, used to gather important clues to the patient's condition and response to treatment. The reduced number of RNs, meanwhile, became responsible for the care of a larger number of patients, while also supervising the care activities of a growing number of nurses' aides, who deliver care at the bedside but lack the skills or the knowledge necessary to recognize, correctly interpret, or communicate vital information about patients. Requiring this information to do their jobs of planning and evaluating care, RNs still needed time—a scarce commodity given RNs' new workloads—with patients to gather this information.

Individually, the nurses in this study shouldered the cost of struggling to deliver the care they deemed necessary. To recover what they considered necessary time with patients, the nurses at BIDMC sped up their work or worked overtime. Dedicated, busy nurses took no time to look after themselves—to eat or even to use the restroom. To protect patient health, nurses paid with their own health and well-being. Many showed signs of burnout from prolonged work speed-up and the frustration and effort of circumventing dysfunctional or inadequate hospital systems.

Many contemplated leaving the nursing profession. Others found it necessary to reduce their hours by becoming part-time or per diem workers.

Despite repeated efforts to bring these new facts of nurses' work life to the attention of administrators, the hospital leadership did not recognize nurses' Herculean efforts to maintain the level of care provided to patients. Confronted with these accounts, they likely saw nurses' efforts as unnecessary, further proof of an unwillingness to accept reasonable but more efficient care standards. Throughout my study, the hospital leadership insisted that nurses' claims of threats to care quality veiled attempts to protect the professional status nurses enjoyed in Beth Israel's glory days. Without glaring evidence of patient dissatisfaction or morbidity, administrators denied that care had been compromised. In management's view, nurses' complaints about time with patients were a matter of their own satisfaction, not patient safety; nurses wanted to protect their autonomy and control over the organization and over patient care. Administrators perceived such self-interested resistance as an obstruction to efficiency and the hospital's attempts to reduce its operating deficit.

In fact, the hospital leadership actively sought to gain greater control over nursing practice by reducing nurses' professional status and influence in the organization. The hospital leadership pushed out the nurse administrators who had led the hospital to international prominence. They broke apart the Nursing Department, distributing nurses to other departments throughout the hospital and making a large portion of nurses subordinate, not to another nurse or health care professional, but to nonclinical managers. Finally, they stripped nurses of their influence over hospital decision making by removing their seat at the executive table through the elimination of the Vice President of Nursing position. Thus, BIDMC joined the ranks of many other hospitals in the late 1990s: While the head of nursing retained a seat at the executive table, it was as the representative of "patient care services" and not of nursing alone (Clifford 1998). Nursing at BIDMC lost its voice as a separate and distinct professional discipline and its power in shaping organizational decisions and policies.

With news stories from across the country reporting clashes between nurses and administrators, it is clear that the conflict between the nurses and administrators at BIDMC goes beyond a local story about changes to a famous model of professional nursing. The drama at Beth Israel seems to be playing out at hospitals across the country, with nurses, their professional organizations, and their unions complaining about not having enough time or support to care for patients. Nurses in several states orchestrated demonstrations and strikes to emphasize work conditions they consider unsafe for both nurses and patients.[6] Some administrators claim that nurses—and particularly their unions—exaggerate the occasional horror story to generate public sympathy and support in labor negotiations with hospitals. These administrators denied problems in their own hospitals and suggested that the clamor disguised the real issue, which is not patient safety, but nurses' fears for their jobs or desire for higher salaries. In short, these administrators suggested that nurses used the language of patient risk to increase their control over organizational policies and practices, not to communicate a real threat to the quality of care.

Similarly, BIDMC's leadership approached nurses' concerns as an either-or proposition. Either nurses were concerned about their own professional status, autonomy, and control, or they were concerned about patient safety and care quality. However, this distinction is meaningless because the issues of nurses' status, autonomy, and control are closely related both to nurses' professional satisfaction and to quality of patient care.

Led by Linda Aiken, a team of researchers from the University of Pennsylvania conducted a series of studies that demonstrate the importance of status, autonomy, and control both for nurses' and patients' well-being. In 1994, Aiken, Smith, and Lake found lower Medicare mortality rates "in a group of hospitals characterized by nurses as being good places to work" (772), Beth Israel among them. Staffing levels and the educational credentials of the nurses could not explain away differences in the number of

[6] A number of news articles in 1999, the year I performed my research, covered conflicts between nurses and hospitals in states across the country, including Massachusetts (Dolores Kong, "Boston-Area Nurses to Join Nationwide Protest over Staffing Levels," *Boston Globe,* 4 Nov. 1999), California (Patrick S. Pemberton, "San Luis Obispo, Calif., Nurses Picket Medical Center," *Tribune,* 11 Sept. 1999), Rhode Island (Brian C. Jones, "Providence, R.I., Hospital Union Protests Nursing Changes," *Providence Journal-Bulletin,* 25 June 1999), North Carolina (Alan Wolf, "Nurses at Durham, N.C., Hospital Consider Unionizing," 19 Feb. 2000), and Alaska (Eve Rose, "Anchorage, Alaska, Hospital's Nurses Are Set to Strike," *Anchorage Daily News,* 4 Apr. 1999). Nurses claimed that concerns over staffing and the quality of patient care led to their protests. This list is in no way exhaustive.

patient deaths. Rather, the results indicate a larger story in which the organization of nurses' work contributes to better patient outcomes. In this and later research they identify the organizational features that both enhance nurses' satisfaction and improve patient outcomes: nurses' status and representation in the hospital, their control over the resources required to perform their work, their autonomy in decisions about how to care for patients, and their teamwork and collegiality with physicians. The researchers found that these organizational arrangements "and their resulting impact on nurses' behaviors on behalf of patients" enhance patient outcomes (Aiken, Smith, and Lake 1994:783; Aiken et al. 1999) and reduce nurses' burnout (Aiken and Sloane 1997a).

Aiken and her colleagues examine how organizational structure influences outcomes for both nurses and patients by creating a more or less supportive environment for nursing care (Aiken and Sloane 1997a; Aiken and Sloane 1997b; Aiken, Sloane, and Lake 1997; Aiken, Smith, and Lake, 1994; Aiken, Sochalski, and Lake, 1997). They identify dedicated AIDS units and magnet hospitals, for example, as structures that promote more supportive contexts for nursing care. Dedicated AIDS units, due to the complex, chronic, and fatal nature of the illness treated and the opportunities for nurses to specialize in its treatment, tend to support favorable working conditions, even when the arrangement of unspecialized units in the same hospital do not (Aiken and Sloane 1997b). Similarly, magnet hospitals, hospitals that embody a set of organizational attributes that nurses find desirable (Aiken, Smith, and Lake 1994: 771), prioritize nursing; for example, representatives of nursing may participate at the highest levels of decision making within the institution. The values and structures in place in magnet hospitals promote a favorable context for nursing care on units, specialized or not, throughout the hospital.

Restructuring could create fluctuations and changes in these important organizational arrangements—nurses' status, their control over the practice environment, their autonomy, and their relationships with physicians—both throughout the institution and within individual units. That BIDMC did not bother to apply to the American Nurses Credentialing Center for recognition as a magnet hospital—one of Beth Israel's distinguishing features—demonstrates just how susceptible to disruption these arrangements are. Such fluctuations and changes could have ramifications not just for individual nurses' satisfaction and burnout rate but also for the quality of care patients receive.

In general, frontline employees bear the brunt of any restructuring effort. Not only must they carry out and adjust to any changes, but they must do so while continuing to perform the work of the organization. Yet we know little about how restructuring alters the organizational arrangements that affect employees' satisfaction, motivation, or performance.

With the assumption that happy employees are also productive employees, a large body of research focuses on carefully planned restructuring strategies (such as job redesign and participation in decision making) that are specifically chosen and designed to humanize the workplace and to promote positive attitudes and behavior among employees. However, studies of this type of planned restructuring yield conflicting results about the effects on employees (see meta-analyses: Guzzo, Jette, and Katzell 1985; Kelly 1992; Miller and Monge 1986; Neuman, Edwards, and Raju 1989; Robertson, Roberts, and Porras 1993; Spector 1986; Wagner 1994; Wagner and Gooding 1987). One reason for these conflicting results is that this research often neglects to assess or report how restructuring actually changed organizational arrangements that influence employees' attitudes and behaviors. Much of it focuses instead on the changes expected by researchers or managers. In complex organizations, however, expected changes may bear little resemblance to actual changes. Even when restructuring goes according to plan, the results may nonetheless be unexpected and even unwelcome.

The issue of examining actual, rather than anticipated, changes from restructuring grows even more salient in the case of strategies chosen not for their effect on employees but for their effect on an organization's finances or performance—for example, mergers or budget reductions. These strategies often entail far-reaching changes to employees' daily work lives—such as changes in the way their work is done, expanded job demands and responsibilities, and changes in their employment status and their pool of coworkers. However, these changes and their effects may not even enter into the decision process in choosing and implementing a strategy. The question of how these strategies change organizational arrangements that affect employees' ability and desire to do their work has gone largely unasked and unanswered. Only a handful of studies have looked at the effect of this type of restructuring on employees. This book is one of the few that addresses the impact in a health care setting.

This book examines how restructuring at BIDMC produced the conditions that made highly educated and skilled nurses question their desire to stay in nursing and their ability to provide good care. The case presented in this book provides insight into the factors detracting from the nursing profession's recruitment and retention of nurses.

Nurses constitute the largest single group of health professionals, and most nurses work in hospitals. Moreover, "[n]urses are the cornerstone of the professional surveillance system in hospitals because they are the only health care professionals at the bedside around the clock" (Aiken, Sochalski, and Lake 1997:NS16). Nurses provide the front line of care in hospital settings and have the most contact with hospital patients as well as the most direct impact on care received. To the extent that changes in organizational arrangements impair nurses' motivation, satisfaction, or performance, adverse outcomes, mortality, and discomfort may all increase for hospital patients.

Surprisingly, the effect of organizational restructuring on nurses and their work has received little public attention. But, I contend, it is no accident that the worst nursing shortage in our nation's history follows on the heels of unprecedented restructuring in the health care industry. While cyclical over- and undersupply of nurses is nothing new, this nursing shortage differs due to a combination of factors. This time around, the nursing shortage involves a sharp increase in demand in tandem with a decrease in supply. The average age among RNs is forty-five. Many plan to retire in the next several years, just as the baby boomers' consumption of health care services is expected to increase (Bednash 2000). There are not enough new RNs in the pipeline. Nursing school admissions fall yearly, and there are few RNs in the eighteen- to twenty-seven-year-old age range (Buerhaus, Staiger, and Auerbach 2000). Hospitals claim that they already feel the shortage and are having trouble attracting and retaining nurses. Unfilled nursing positions account for approximately 75 percent of hospital job vacancies. Moreover, a disturbing number of RNs are leaving the profession. A recent study of 43,329 RNs in Pennsylvania reported that 22 percent planned to leave nursing (Aiken et al. 2001). Hospital restructuring drove many experienced nurses away from the bedside and may have scared off potential new recruits.

Lawmakers, hospitals, and nurses' groups seek solutions to the problems of retaining and attracting nurses. A number of states have introduced legislation to ban mandatory overtime, and others are considering mandating minimum nurse-staffing ratios. The American Nurses Association has requested more money from the government for recruitment and education of new nurses. While many of these solutions address nurses' most immediate complaints, they may only treat symptoms rather than the underlying disease. The problem is that hospital restructuring has fundamentally changed organizational arrangements that shape nurses' daily work lives and what it means to be a nurse.

In *Beyond Caring* (1996), Daniel Chambliss identifies three core features of nurses' work, which he labels "missions": "The hospital nurse is expected, and typically expects herself, to be simultaneously (1) a caring individual, (2) a professional, and (3) a relatively subordinate member of the organization" (62). For nurses, caring involves working face to face with patients for an extended amount of time, a condition that gives nurses claims to special kinds of knowledge about patients (Anspach 1996; Chambliss 1996). It includes treating patients as human beings, not just diseases or ailments that need to be cured. The second mission, being professional, emphasizes that caring is a job that nurses must perform regardless of the situation or the characteristics of their patient. Professionalism requires that caring be performed with special competence, a bringing to bear of clinical expertise and judgment even under pressure and time constraints. For nurses, being a professional signifies a claim to special status and respect, "polite treatment by doctors, the listening ear of administrators, the respect of outsiders" (Chambliss 1996:71). The third mission, subordination, concerns the context of nurses' employment in organizations and their lesser status in comparison to the medical profession. Nurses are simultaneously subordinate to the administrators in the organizations in which they work and to the doctors whose orders they carry out. Even though nurses may exercise professional judgment, their daily work is shaped and guided by others. Together these three missions define what nurses' work is (caring), how they perform it (as professionals), and under what constraints (as subordinates to hospital administrators and to doctors). These three missions produce some of the conflicts inherent in being a nurse: "The directives conflict: be caring and yet be professional, be subordinate and yet responsible, be diffusely accountable for a patient's well-being and yet oriented to the hospital as an economic employer" (Chambliss 1996:62).

While these conflicts have long plagued nursing, hospital cost-cutting and downsizing in the late 1990s increased the dissonance among these aspects of nurses' work. In particular, hospital restructuring devalued the caring aspects of nurses' role, strained their ability to act as professionals, and emphasized their subordination to institutions that find it necessary to emphasize margin over mission. In the process, nursing, which became less attractive once women were liberated to enter male professions, has become even less attractive. But the tensions among these three aspects of the nurse's role are not unique to nursing; the same conflicts exist for all of the caring professions employed in bureaucratic organizations. To the extent that the shifted balance among nurses' caring, professionalism, and subordination to their hospital employers has made nursing less attractive, this is a cautionary tale for other caring professions employed by resource-strapped organizations, such as doctors, social workers, and teachers.

This book presents an in-depth view of changes that affected nurses at Beth Israel Deaconess Medical Center from January to September 1999. The book reports the findings gathered during nine months of intensive field research at the hospital. During those nine months, I shadowed nurses on six different units that served the adult medical-surgical population. I attended staff meetings, interviewed nurses and administrators, held focus groups with floor nurses, distributed surveys, and studied internal hospital reports and documents. I collected data about how organizational arrangements had changed and how nurses' work had changed as a result. I attended to the issues of power and control and their relationship to nurses' ability to perform their work.

In Chapter 2, I place BIDMC's Code Green and selected solutions in the context of changes in the hospital industry. Chapter 3 considers the very different nursing models in use at the two premerger hospitals and the way changes at BIDMC undermined nurses' continued use of these models to deliver patient care. The mistaken assumptions that led to the view of nurses as obstacles to restructuring and ultimately to the dismantling of the Nursing Department are described in Chapter 4. Using the case of the Emergency Department, Chapter 5 examines the effects of ongoing power conflicts—a vestige of the bungled merger—on nurses' ability to provide care to patients. The consolidation of the Cardiothoracic Unit illustrates, in Chapter 6, the impact of physicians' conflicts with each other on the relationships between doctors and nurses and on nurses' control over their own practice. Through an analysis of the assumptions used to calculate the new nurse-staffing levels on the inpatient units, Chapter 7 discusses nurses' perception that they did not have enough time to provide what they considered safe care to patients. Chapter 8 explores the dispute between nurses and administrators over whether restructuring compromised the quality of care at BIDMC. Chapter 9, the conclusion, evaluates the restructuring strategies that BIDMC pursued, the effects on nurses' roles as caring and professional, and the implications for the future nursing workforce.

1

A Troubled Hospital

In 1995, Mitchell Rabkin recognized that the hospital he had headed since 1966 now faced some serious problems. Quickly approaching retirement, this icon in the Massachusetts medical community needed to think about how to safeguard his hospital's commitment to its patients and employees and still compete in an increasingly hostile, competitive medical marketplace. With Vice President of Nursing Joyce Clifford, Rabkin had transformed this Jewish community hospital into one of the best-known medical research and teaching institutions in the world. Beth Israel Hospital, fondly known as "Harvard with a Heart," stood out among the other Harvard teaching hospitals for its human touch. The hospital was a friendly place both to its patients and its employees. *Modern Healthcare* had listed Beth Israel among the top one hundred hospitals in the country, while *Working Mothers Magazine* recognized the hospital as one of the country's best workplaces for women.[1] Even with this focus on the human factor, Rabkin ran a tight ship. Despite ferocious cost-cutting on the part of Massachusetts insurers, Beth Israel operated in the black. Moreover, a 1994 William M. Mercer Analysis judged the hospital to be the most efficient of Boston's six largest teaching hospitals.[2] Despite these considerable achievements, the hospital was beginning to strain under the pressures in the health care market. It needed to take dramatic action to ensure its survival.

[1] Alex Pham, "Human Touch at the Top: Amid Merger Mania Beth Israel Chief Takes Time to Chat with Patient and Pick Up Litter," *Boston Globe*, 7 Mar. 1995, Economy 39.
[2] Ibid.

The conditions that necessitated dramatic action were not unique to Beth Israel Hospital or to the Massachusetts health care market. The pressures that Beth Israel faced and the choices its leadership made in response reflect broader trends in the U.S. hospital industry. To understand what happened to nursing at Beth Israel, we have to understand how the context in which nursing was practiced dramatically shifted in the mid-1990s.

Changes in the Hospital Industry

Over the past few decades there have been sweeping changes in the U.S. health care system. Over the last two decades, both public and private purchasers of health care services have pressured hospitals to contain their cost growth. The historical roots of these trends relate to the consolidation of purchasers of health care services. Increasingly, the purchasing of health insurance and health services, traditionally an individual affair, is now conducted by collective purchasers. This change began in the public sector in 1965 with the advent of Medicare and Medicaid. Consolidation also took place in the private sector through growth of the health insurance industry as it became increasingly common for employers to purchase group insurance to provide health benefits to employees (Starr 1982). By removing payment responsibility from individual consumers of health services, this growth of public and private health insurance increased access to and demand for health services. Meanwhile, technological advances improved or created the ability to perform new procedures and treatments and further fueled demand. This market environment spurred rapid increases in national health care spending.

At their inception, Medicare and Medicaid adopted generous payment policies to encourage physicians and hospitals to accept Medicare and Medicaid patients (Starr 1982). These programs provided fee-for-service payment for health care. This system encouraged hospitals and physicians to perform numerous services because they received payment for each service rendered (Robinson and Casalino 1996). This payment system provided little incentive for hospitals to scrutinize practice, to increase efficiency, or to limit costs. Charges for services varied widely from hospital to hospital and region to region. The federal government, footing the bill, attempted to control escalating cost growth in these public programs during the 1970s. In large part due to the incentives built into the reimbursement system, these efforts proved ineffective.

In 1983 the federal government attempted to rein in its Medicare outlays for hospital services by changing these incentives through introduction of a prospective payment system. Under prospective payment, Medicare paid predetermined amounts for various hospital services. Costs were determined not by individual hospitals but through a calculation that adjusted costs based, among other criteria, on region and type of hospital. Since Medicare accounts for almost 40 percent of hospital revenues, the program had considerable potential to move the hospital industry toward greater efficiency (PROPAC 1997). Instead, the costs for hospital services continued to rise, and Medicare payments fell below the costs of services (Guterman, Ashby, and Greene 1996). Rather than pursue greater efficiency, hospitals tended to shift costs onto private payers (Guterman, Ashby, and Greene 1996).

The employers who pay for health care in the U.S. employment-based system soon followed the government's example and also sought to reduce cost growth. Managed care was chosen as the primary means for changing physician and hospital behavior. It substituted fee-for-service with payment systems that increased physician and hospital accountability and risk (PROPAC 1997) and introduced insurance company micromanagement of discrete services. Private insurers began to take a more active role in managing hospital care. They refused payment for services deemed unnecessary and, in some cases, capped total payments. With the number of individuals in managed care plans growing, the largest health plans could effectively use their leverage to negotiate favorable contracts with hospitals. Furthermore, new technologies made it possible to perform many inpatient procedures on an outpatient basis. Hospitals experienced competition from freestanding facilities to perform these services (Kuttner 1999). Large insurers pressured hospitals into deep discounts on services by threatening to take their business elsewhere.

Until the late 1990s most hospitals were able to manage cost-cutting pressures and still retain profit margins. Mounting cost-containment pressure from the private sector limited hospitals' ability to shift costs to the private sector for uncompensated and underfunded care. Consequently, hospitals sought greater efficiency (Guterman, Ashby, and Greene 1996). In the 1990s, as hospitals became more efficient, Medicare payments once again exceeded costs (Levit et al. 1998). The relationship of private and public payers reversed (Levit et al. 2000; PROPAC 1997), and the public sector's comparatively generous payments now subsidized the deep discounts demanded by the private sector.

The Balanced Budget Act (BBA) of 1997 moved to change this arrangement. The BBA mandated reduction of Medicare expenditures by $115 billion over five years, including a $17 billion reduction in projected Medicare hospital payments (Kuttner 1999). This legislation effectively removed the cushion for hospitals that depended on Medicare payments to cover their cost shortfall from managed care and other insurance contracts. Reports of losses in the millions of dollars for fiscal year 1999 reveal how close to the bone hospital margins have been cut. As a result, some of the BBA Medicare payment reductions have been reversed or postponed (Hallam 1999), and further rollbacks are being considered (Levit et al. 2000).

Teaching hospitals and hospitals serving poorer communities have been hard hit by the market crunch. These hospitals face higher costs to treat patients. These costs include teaching, research, treating more acute cases, and caring for the poor (Blumenthal and Meyer 1996; Reuter and Gaskin 1997). These additional costs impede these hospitals' ability to compete for managed care contracts on price (Reuter and Gaskin 1997). For example, academic health centers charge between 15 percent and 35 percent more per inpatient admission (adjusted for case-mix) than their community hospital competitors (Blumenthal and Meyer 1996). Medicare payments subsidize the added costs of these hospitals' teaching and social missions (Blumenthal and Meyer 1996). But the BBA Medicare payment reductions have sent many of these institutions into financial crisis.

Strong lobbying by teaching and other hospitals convinced Congress that the cuts were more draconian than intended, and hospitals received a billion-dollar "giveback" to offset some of the burden.[3] However, this

[3] "Teaching Hospitals: Hit Hard by Budget Cuts," *American Health Line,* 28 Apr. 1999; Kristen Hallam, "Givebacks; Healthcare Wins on Medicare, Wants More," *Modern Healthcare,* 29 Nov. 1999; "Boston Teaching Hospitals Fight the Good Fight," *American Health Line,* 14 Oct. 1999; "New HCIA Data Show BBA Cuts May Squeeze Hospital Finances More Than An-

temporary reprieve did nothing to solve the larger issues of how hospitals might come out of Code Green while balancing cost-containment and social mission. Moreover, it came too late to offset the effects of the kinds of cost-cutting strategies employed by hospitals to deal with the pressures of managed care.

Hospitals' Search for Solutions

As soon as managed care became the nation's de facto health care policy, hospitals responded to market pressures with tactics to manage their internal operations and external environment. In the 1990s, hospitals devised a number of strategies to wring cost reductions out of their internal operations. Since labor costs (salaries, wages, and benefits) eat the largest chunk of a hospital's budget, over one-half on average (PROPAC 1997; Robertson, Dowd, and Hassan 1997), the most popular strategies target these costs. From 1981 through 1993, overall hospital employment increased by 11.3 percent, controlling for increased patient volume and acuity (Aiken, Sochalski, and Anderson 1996). In 1994, this trend began to reverse, with the number of hospital employees decreasing even as patient admissions increased (PROPAC 1997). Therefore, hospitals have placed greater productivity demands on each employee. Popular labor-cutting strategies included changing skill mix by introducing a larger proportion of assistants and unlicensed personnel and reducing the number of registered nurses, lowering staff-to-patient ratios, and cross-training staff to take on more functions (Shindul-Rothschild, Berry, and Long-Middleton 1996). At the same time, hospitals have restrained annual increases in employees' compensation relative to the rest of the economy (PROPAC 1997).

In addition to their efforts to save money, hospitals also pursued strategies to make more money. One common strategy hospitals used was to shift many of their services from an inpatient to an outpatient basis (Levit et al. 1998). Because outpatient procedures generally cost less than inpatient, private insurers under managed care favor ambulatory surgery, home care, and

---

ticipated," *Health Management Technology,* Sept. 1999; "HCIA: BBA Impact on Hospitals 'Bleaker' Than Imagined," *American Health Line,* 5 Oct. 1999.

hospice care (Kuttner 1999; Robinson and Casalino 1996). Hospitals responded to this market by offering a greater range of outpatient services and shifting inpatient services to an outpatient basis where possible. Additionally, hospitals shortened the length of stay by sending patients to nursing homes, hospice care, rehabilitation facilities, or home or even hotels once insurers, hospitals, and doctors deemed they no longer required the more intense monitoring available in hospital inpatient facilities. Medicare prospective payment further encouraged this trend. Medicare reimbursement for outpatient care may be obtained in addition to inpatient care reimbursement: Hospitals received the same prospective payment for caring for a patient for fewer days, thereby improving profit margin, while patients received coverage for continued care in another facility.

As a result of this move away from inpatient services, the number of outpatient visits nearly doubled between 1983 and 1998, increasing from 273,168 to 520,600 visits a year in community hospitals (American Hospital Association 1999). In contrast, the number of inpatient visits remained relatively steady, falling from 38,887 to 33,624 visits per year in community hospitals (American Hospital Association 1999). The percentage of hospital revenue from outpatient services increased from 14.4 percent to 30.1 percent between 1984 and 1996. The percentage of hospital revenue from inpatient services declined from 81.3 percent to 64 percent, but the total volume of hospital services continued to grow (PROPAC 1997).

In tandem with this shift to outpatient services, the average length of stay shortened, falling steadily since 1983 (PROPAC 1997). The average length of stay in U.S. hospitals decreased by almost two full days, from 7.2 days in 1981 to 5.5 days in 1996, and continues to fall (American Hospital Association 1999; Levit et al. 2000; PROPAC 1997).

This transition toward greater outpatient services created serious challenges for hospitals while promising increased revenue. While outpatient services might be less expensive for hospitals to deliver, they often required construction of new facilities, investment in new equipment, and hiring and recruitment of qualified staff. This spending could negate gains in the payment-to-cost margin (Greene 1992). Additionally, the rise of postacute care services meant that only the sickest patients required inpatient hospitalization. As a result, the average medical-surgical patients in the 1990s were as acutely ill as critical care patients in the 1980s (Curtin and Simpson 2000). Moreover, these patients would be discharged as soon as they required less intensive care. These two trends, higher patient acuity and shortened length of stay, together and individually, increased the workload per patient day at a time when many hospitals were also decreasing their labor force. These trends concentrated a group of more demanding patients at the time when they needed the most care in hospitals in which employees were already being asked to provide care with less help.

Although the shift to greater outpatient care profited hospitals in some ways, it also left them with an oversupply of beds (Kuttner 1999). In response, many hospitals formed organized delivery systems or integrated networks (American Hospital Association 1999; Duke 1996; Levit et al. 1998), vertically integrating with both primary care and postacute care providers. Because physicians often play an active role in determining where their patients will be treated, partnering with primary care physicians provided hospitals with a greater competitive edge in capturing business (Duke 1996). Hospitals also sought access to revenue from postacute care services and pursued integration with postacute care organizations (e.g., nursing homes, rehabilitation facilities, home care, and hospice care) or converted former inpatient units to postacute care facilities. In the early 1990s, integration with primary and postacute care providers took the form of acquisition. In the latter half of the decade "virtual" integration, through exclusive contracts or strategic alliances, became more prevalent (Shortell et al. 1997). Through virtual and actual integration hospitals hoped to gain a greater competitive advantage in negotiating and competing for managed care contracts (Levit et al. 2000) and in ensuring a steady stream of patients from physician referrals.

Hospitals also pursued relationships with other hospitals in response to cost pressures and overcapacity (Duke 1996; Levit et al. 2000). These horizontal mergers and alliances served a number of different purposes depending on the relationships among the hospitals, but, in general, this strategy served one of two purposes: not "managing competition" but the elimination of the competition or the expansion of the hospital network to gain a monopolistic edge (Bogue et al. 1995). These strategies enabled hospitals to pool their market share, making the merged entity a larger competitor in the local market.

Hospitals serving noncompeting locales often formed multihospital networks. Participation in multihospital networks generates greater bargaining power with managed care companies due to the ability to provide multiple services in a variety of locations (Dranove, Durkac, and Shanley 1996). For small hospitals, these networks might mean a greater portfolio of services to help attract managed care contracts. Network expansion could shift the balance of power in negotiations with managed care companies that needed access to particular hospitals in the network in order to offer a full range of services to their customers (Barro and Cutler 1997).

In the merger mania that swept the hospital industry in the 1990s, hospitals competing in close proximity have tended to enter mergers. Between 1990 and 1996, 176 hospital mergers took place in the United States—more than in the entire previous decade (Spang, Bazzoli, and Arnould 2001). These mergers resulted in the closing of one of the hospitals, division of specialty functions between the hospitals involved, or, less commonly, parallel operations but with an integration of administrative functions (Barro and Cutler 1997). Not only did these mergers neutralize a rival hospital, but they promised hospitals cost-savings from realization of economies of scale. By merging with other institutions, hospitals hoped to expand their market share, gain stronger footing with managed care companies, and more easily access a stable customer base (Brazzoli et al. 2002; Bogue et al. 1995; Dranove, Durkac, and Shanley 1996).

The Beth Israel–Deaconess Merger: A Problematic Solution

Massachusetts General Hospital and Brigham and Women's Hospital, the two largest of the Harvard teaching hospitals, took the Boston medical scene by surprise when they announced their merger in 1993. Full-page ads in the *Boston Globe* and the *New York Times* among others, announced that these titans of Massachusetts medicine created Partners HealthCare Inc. This new giant health care network—with 12,000 employees, 2,100 beds, and nearly 4,000 physicians[4]—boasted it would meet all of the med-

[4] Alex Pham, "Beth Israel, Deaconess Announce Merger Plan," *Boston Globe,* 24 Feb. 1996, Metro/Region 1.

ical needs from primary care to hospitalization of a majority of Boston-area residents. This formidable competitor threatened to gobble up market share and starve out Beth Israel along with the other local hospitals. The situation required action. Rabkin and the hospital board believed that if Beth Israel wanted to remain a player in this market, it needed to team with another institution.

In 1996 Beth Israel Hospital announced it would join forces with New England Deaconess Hospital, its neighbor across the street. Individually the two hospitals had been losing market share to Partners HealthCare.[5] Both hospitals considered the union a necessary step to compete and ultimately thrive in the Massachusetts health care market. The Deaconess had already merged with four community hospitals to form Pathways Health Network. But the five hospitals combined were only a little bigger than Beth Israel in terms of total revenues, assets, and the number of employees.[6] Pathways perceived that it needed the greater clout, prestige, and referral base that affiliation with a strong Boston teaching hospital could provide.[7] Together with Mount Auburn Hospital in Cambridge, these hospitals formed CareGroup, a network second in size only to Partners Healthcare.

The newly formed Beth Israel Deaconess Medical Center (BIDMC) would be CareGroup network's flagship hospital, its crown jewel, with 1,257 physicians, 7,660 employees, and nearly $1 billion in annual revenue.[8] Together these CareGroup hospitals would play David to the behemoth Goliath that was Partners Healthcare. Alone they could not compete, but together, the hospitals thought, they might reclaim some of the market share now hoarded by Partners.

Unlike the Partners' merger that joined administrative functions only, the Beth Israel–Deaconess merger required full integration and consolidation of the two hospitals. The two hospitals stood to realize a strong economic advantage—savings of millions of dollars—by combining over-

[5] Alex Pham. "Beth Israel, Deaconess Announce Merger Plan," *Boston Globe,* 24 Feb. 1996, Metro/Region 1.

[6] Alex Pham and Charles Stein, "Deaconess, Beth Israel Study Alliance; Both Failed to Close Deals with Other Hospitals in 1995," *Boston Globe,* 19 Jan. 1996.

[7] Alex Pham, "Mt. Auburn Set to Merge With Hospitals; Union Would Form $1b Health Care Network," *Boston Globe,* 12 Mar. 1996.

[8] Alex Pham, "Beth Israel, Deaconess Announce Merger Plan," *Boston Globe,* 24 Feb. 1996, Metro/Region 1.

lapping departments and sharing administrative expenses.[9] They planned to merge the hospital boards as well as all clinical and administrative functions. The press heralded this dramatic change in management with optimistic newspaper reports touting the advantages of the planned combination. Beth Israel offered large cash reserves and a strong obstetrics service, while Deaconess brought strong programs in gastroenterology and cardiology to the marriage.[10]

Though hopes were high, the merger was also a risky proposition. Although it seemed Beth Israel's best chance to remain a strong institution, the merger would change the hospital. The merged entity would no longer be Beth Israel Hospital, but something different. Perhaps the best of the two hospitals, perhaps the best of neither.

Three years after the merger, the gamble had not paid off. Despite the initial optimism, the Beth Israel–Deaconess merger did not deliver on its financial promise and even weakened the hospital's situation.

Integration and consolidation of the two neighboring hospitals had progressed little by 1999, when I conducted my field research. Even making allowances for the sheer logistical difficulty involved in closing down hospital facilities and moving whole departments, the process proved more difficult than initially anticipated.[11] Duplications in administrative positions and medical and surgical specialties burdened the hospital with greater expenses than planned. Under these circumstances, BIDMC had yet to realize any of the promised financial returns from the merger.

The honeymoon between Beth Israel and the Deaconess hospitals had long been over when my fieldwork began at BIDMC in 1999. Prominent surgeons and physicians, angry at the way the merger had been handled or displeased with new arrangements, left their positions at the hospital, draining its prestige. In May 1998, forty contract anesthesiologists serving the Deaconess campus quit en masse in response to a contract renewal offer deemed "unpalatable."[12] This left the anesthesiologists on the Beth Is-

[9] Ibid.

[10] Ibid.; Alex Pham and Charles Stein, "Deaconess, Beth Israel Study Alliance; Both Failed to Close Deals With Other Hospitals in 1995," *Boston Globe,* 19 January 1996.

[11] Richard Saltus and Alex Pham, "BI Deaconess Still Feeling Merger Pain: Medical Center Morale, Reputation Suffer," *Boston Globe,* 28 Jan. 1999.

[12] Michael Lasalandra, "Deaths May Be Symptom of Medical Merger-Mania," *Boston Herald,* 7 June 1998.

rael campus to cover both hospitals. Afterward, four unexpected surgical deaths occurred at the hospital. The Department of Public Health investigated the connection to the anesthesiology staffing crisis.[13] Although no evidence was found to substantiate a link between the staffing shortage and the deaths, BIDMC suffered negative publicity. Prompted by events at BIDMC, the *Boston Herald* published an article with the headline "Deaths May Be Symptom of Medical Merger-Mania."[14] The report suggested that financially motivated mergers throughout the hospital industry have not been evaluated for safety and efficacy. Officials at BIDMC felt that the Boston-area papers took a heavy-handed approach in this and other articles and misrepresented events. Rumors about a "deep throat" in the organization abounded. Staff from both hospitals were disheartened by the bad press, and each side blamed the other for the tarnish on the hospital's sterling reputation.

The hospitals remained two distinct entities. Although the hospitals neighbored one another, moving between them required walking two or three blocks outside. Walking from one end of the campus to the other took more than twenty minutes. This distance proved a challenge for staff to get back and forth for meetings or to see patients, and it was especially inconvenient during the inclement New England winter. In addition to the geographical distinctness, each campus had its own way of doing things: different paperwork, computer systems, and models of care delivery. These differences, some trivial, made it difficult for clinical staff to move back and forth across the campuses as needed.

In observations and interviews, a frustrated staff warned that these slight variations could hinder patient care. In an often-repeated example, the color used to flag physician orders needing to be filled differed on the two campuses, with the color used on one campus meaningless on the other. If a Deaconess doctor visiting the Beth Israel campus used the usual Deaconess color to flag orders, the orders would be ignored. In telling the story, staff members cautioned that this innocent mistake could delay patient care and potentially prove harmful. This trivial decision of which colors to use for flagging orders—a decision that could have been made with

[13] Ibid.; Michael Lasalandra, "Medical Alert; State Asked to Probe Beth Israel Deaconess After 4 Deaths," *Boston Herald,* 22 July 1998.

[14] Lasalandra, *Boston Herald,* 7 June 1998.

a coin toss—took two years to make. Moreover, once it was made, the Deaconess staff griped that their color system had not been chosen. With growing anger, they complained that they were being forced to do everything the Beth Israel way.

Power Struggles and Merger Disappointments

The issue of the color of the flags used on charts signaled a far deeper rift that affected every discipline in the hospital, including nursing. That this rift should occur would not surprise anyone who studied the problems of mergers in hospitals or other industries.

A small but growing body of research on the human factor in mergers and acquisitions explores why between two-thirds and three-fourths of mergers—not just in hospitals but in all industries—fail to deliver the financial benefits predicted by rational economic models (Cartwright and Cooper 1993; Marks and Mirvis 1992). The emerging answer is that these models have failed to take into account the human costs and consequences of organizational combinations. The responses of employees left behind to continue operations are crucial to a merger's success (Buono and Bowditch 1989; Buono and Nurick 1992; Cartwright and Cooper 1993; Covin et al. 1996), but the responses tend to be destructive due to merger-related stress, often sparked by culture conflict between the merging organizations (Lubatkin and Lane 1996; Marks and Mirvis 1992).

Cultural clashes between two merging organizations become prominent several months or more after a formal merger due to the difficulties inherent in integrating employees from two different organizations with different styles, approaches, and sometimes missions (Buono and Bowditch 1989). As Mitchell Marks and Philip Mirvis (1992) explain, mergers tend to produce an "us versus them" attitude. As a result, workers feel threatened by the newcomers' beliefs and values about the best way of doing things. Such cultural collisions occur even in mergers between companies that seem to be culturally similar (Cartwright and Cooper 1993).

Research on human factors in mergers and acquisitions attends to culture clashes over the best way of doing things as primary causes of merger failure. However, these clashes are not so much a problem of incompatible cultures as of power relations. Behind these difficulties associated with cultural collisions is a larger sociological story about shifts in power among different constituencies in the merged organization.

Conflicts over power play a central role in the story of restructuring at BIDMC. *Power* is the influence one wields over a situation, "the ability to get things done the way one wants them to be done" (Salancik and Pfeffer 1977:374). Power may be considered as a finite amount, where one person's having power means another person has less. Alternatively, it may be viewed as an expanding amount, which enables many people to be empowered at once. Daniel Katz and Robert Kahn (1978) explain that the amount of power depends on the situation, on whether there is commonality or conflict of interest:

> Let us assume that A and B are working for the same goals, and that A will be influenced by suggestions from B and B by suggestions from A. The total influence exerted is greater than if A had merely given orders to B. And the effective outcome in productivity may well be greater and the return to both members greater. When, however, we are dealing with a conflict of interest and A and B are engaged in a power struggle, then the more A controls a given decision the less power B has. (322)

Katz and Kahn's explanation illustrates how the view of power as finite applies in conflict situations, whereas the view of power as expanding applies in situations of common interest.

Employees coming together in merged organizations view decisions about whose way will be adopted as signals indicating who has power and influence in the new organization. These decisions are perceived as zero-sum games in which there are winners and losers. The source of merger-related stress may lie less in giving up one's favored ways of doing things and more in the feelings of powerlessness associated with not making others do things one's own way.

In the case of the BIDMC merger, parties from both of the premerger hospitals cast decisions about the best way of doing things in the new hospital as power conflicts. In this context of conflict, power became a win-lose proposition. Every decision about how to perform work could be interpreted as a power struggle, in which one side exerted power over the other. This situation rendered some employees powerful and others powerless in decisions. A zero-sum power struggle can have serious consequences when it renders individuals powerless to influence decisions. As Kanter (1977) explains, "When a person's exercise of power is thwarted or blocked, when people are rendered powerless in the larger arena, they may tend to concentrate their power on those over whom they have even a modicum of authority" (189). Such dynamics led managers and employees at the hospital to resist minor, even trivial, changes and to obstruct others in their attempts to get work done.

Emotion-laden discussions about whose way was best clouded efforts to integrate the Beth Israel and Deaconess staffs and campuses. In an interview, a physician astutely commented on the initial expectations that now bogged down the process to integrate ways of doing things on the two campuses: "We all sat around and said that what we are going to do is come together and then from the different ways that everybody does things, we'll pick the best." He portrayed the resulting problem as a fundamental disagreement over how to define "best" in order to identify practices that should be selected: "Nobody ever had the conversation of 'what's best to you? What does best mean to you? . . . Define best and what it looks like.' As it turns out, each of us defines it differently. And then when your best that you choose to run the hospital isn't the same as my best, then I'm angry, because you're not really out to do what's best; you just want to preserve what is yours" (June 1999). Each decision represented an affront to someone's way of doing things. The selection of one way over another came to represent a judgment that one side of the street did something right and the other side did it wrong. Each side fought vigorously to defend and retain its own way of doing things.

Senior administrators observed, in hindsight, that trying to ease into change had been the wrong approach. As one administrator explained, "We tried not to cause harm—for people to feel like they were being neglected or discounted or not considered in the equation. That was a mistake . . . whatever somebody considered to be the way to go should have been done without an effort to preserve the other side. There were two of everything; they weren't going to survive." He compared the BIDMC merger to the Citibank merger in which "7,000 people would lose their jobs. They didn't try to preserve 7,000 people, they didn't even worry about them, and they just got rid of them. . . . In one sense, Citibank probably works better—they don't care. Or, they do care, and they learned that you just do it and get it over with, and everybody starts to then heal" (March 1999). Senior administrators perceived that such unilateral decision making might have limited the conflicts that the merger fueled between managers from the two premerger hospitals; declaring one side powerless at the outset might have avoided the battles to preserve or exercise power that prolonged the change process.

Trying to cater to all of the constituents prolonged the change process and, according to numerous accounts, created unnecessary suffering. However, a hospital is more complex than a bank because decisions may literally be a matter of life and death. Each side thought that their institutional practices prior to the merger served patients' best interest. Regardless of management stance at the outset, it would have been difficult to avoid conflicts over leadership and decision-making styles because staff perceived that so much hung in the balance.

The simmering conflict finally erupted in December 1998. The Deaconess surgeons, upon whom the Deaconess had built its reputation for excellence as a tertiary referral hospital, had grown increasingly dissatisfied and angry with current policies and process. Several prominent Deaconess surgeons demanded that the administration fire the Chief of Surgery, who was a former Beth Israel surgeon. They threatened to leave the hospital if their demand went unmet. This threat reverberated through the rank and file at the Deaconess, who felt that the surgeons' departure would mean the final dismantling of their once-great institution.

In response to this organizational unrest, James Reinertsen, CEO of CareGroup, the parent company of BIDMC, delivered a landmark address to the medical staff in an emergency meeting on 23 December 1998. His speech to the doctors and nurses in attendance addressed the rift between the staff from the former hospitals: "I personally have become extremely distressed by . . . the fighting in the cockpit. . . . It's quite analogous to the pilot and the copilot and the navigator fighting at the front of the airplane while passengers are being flown. It's unseemly and puts patients at risk, and it must stop. My diagnosis is quite simple. I think we have badly bungled this merger."[15]

Reinertsen described the initial optimism and enthusiasm that the merger "would create the single most powerful medical-surgical hospital in the area." He then asked how since the merger these views had transformed into "pessimism, and anger, and despair, and . . . almost hatred." His answer pointed to "a number of one-sided appointments to a lot of managerial and clinical positions" that favored candidates from the former Beth Israel: "[The appointments may] have all been done individually on the merits, but that was a signal that was not very well received politically and started to cause . . . a lot of unintended victims to be created."

In this speech, Reinertsen, who never worked at either of the premerger hospitals, validated the bitterness brewing among the Deaconess staff. Although on paper the combination of the two hospitals had been a merger and not an acquisition, staff from the Deaconess experienced the merger as a takeover. They perceived that their hospital, only one-third the size of Beth Israel, had been swallowed up by its larger neighbor. Moreover, the composition of the new hospital's leadership reinforced the takeover perception: Deaconess administrators received second-string appointments at every step in the merger process. Two years into the merger, three-fourths of the top administrators from the Deaconess had left the organization for positions elsewhere.

A New Way of Working

Reinertsen conveniently laid the blame for the bungled merger at the feet of the Beth Israel leadership, namely Rabkin, whom Reinertsen had recently replaced as the CEO of CareGroup. In Reinertsen's view, when the Beth Israel leadership staged its takeover of the Deaconess, they imposed an inefficient system for decision making. The system had worked under Rabkin's charismatic leadership, but Rabkin had left his post at Beth Israel to become the head of CareGroup after the merger. In his absence, the Beth Israel management style had crippled the hospital in its turn-

[15] James Reinertsen, M.D., address to the medical staff, BIDMC, December 23, 1998. Transcribed from videotape. All of the quotes from Reinertsen in this section are from this source.

around efforts. Reinertsen emphasized that it was time for the BIDMC leadership to adopt a new way of working.

Prior to the merger, the two sets of hospital leaders utilized very different ways of working to solve problems. Beth Israel had a consensus-based decision-making style, whereas Deaconess managers utilized a more data-oriented process. The Beth Israel management style required lengthy discussions and depended on everyone feeling comfortable with a decision before any action could be taken. In the idealized version of this consensus-based process, objections would be grounded in people's expertise and experience. Decisions benefited from everyone's contribution and buy-in. The shared purpose and participation in the decision-making process worked to empower everyone involved.

However, in the postmerger environment, this decision-making process had broken down. The Beth Israel administrators, who dominated leadership positions in BIDMC, faced much more complex managerial responsibilities. Now that the "family" had grown, Beth Israel's consensus-based process proved too cumbersome to make the many decisions needed to move forward with the merger. Moreover, given the growing merger-related resentments on both sides, joint decisions had become an arena for power contests.

In an interview, an administrator described the way this management style made it difficult for even simple decisions to be made in the new postmerger environment. She explained, "It's sort of like your decision can get stopped anywhere along the line: Just when you think you're all set and everybody is signed off, . . . one administrative person . . . says, 'ugh,' and all the work that's been done doesn't matter. It's not going to happen. That sometimes can happen for darn good reasons, but . . . there were plenty of times where it came where, 'you didn't consult with me.' Now, it's like luck if anything gets pressed through" (March 1999). Pettiness had crept into the process: People would veto plans just because they had not been consulted up front. Some former Deaconess employees even intimated that plans could be rejected just because of who suggested them.

This development was especially troubling in light of the Deaconess management style, which many described as "data-driven." The Deaconess leadership had borrowed from industry an innovative new approach to workforce efficiency and quality insurance. This process, known as total quality management (TQM) or continuous quality improvement (CQI), originated in manufacturing. It involves the use of statistical methods to measure quality and costs and to uncover bottlenecks in the work process. This information is then used to "eliminate redundancies" in production and reengineer the work process (Appelbaum and Batt 1994:90). Eileen Appelbaum and Rosemary Batt explain the TQM process:

> Objective measures of quality become part of employee evaluations. . . . Management information systems transfer data on employee performance to finance departments, where accounting systems incorporate measures of the cost of quality into financial analysis. All employees receive training in quality and customer consciousness, and often in statistical process control as well. The purpose of the training is to "align" the vision of all employees toward a common goal. In this sense, participation is mandatory or expected, rather than voluntary. (1994:90)

In the early 1990s, the Deaconess used this method to streamline its work process and eliminate staff positions and waste as part of a financial turnaround. Their early adoption of this technique placed the hospital on the forefront of innovations in hospital management and streamlining. Employees were trained in how to use data to understand the costs of different work processes and to assess the quality outcomes. In the idealized version of this management style, everyone shared the vision of reducing costs while improving or maintaining quality, and the organization continuously evaluated its processes. Managers from the former Deaconess insisted that under their system it did not matter who you were; power to shape decisions came from having the data to back your ideas.

Beth Israel managers and administrators remained skeptical about the wisdom in relying on data over and against personal judgment and experience. A nurse manager articulated doubts about depending on quantitative data, rather than on people's experience and insight, to make decisions. She explained that at the old Beth Israel, "We got our work done through people. We didn't get our work done through rules and regulations and charts and graphs. You can put anything on paper, and that's what we did with consolidation. . . . You have all these different items that look wonderful on paper, and you sit there, and now it ain't gonna happen" (May 1999). Another nurse manager expressed a commonly held view: "I think in our haste to get problems solved, there's a lot of emphasis now on data. . . . Well, the truth is, data can be cut a lot of different ways. And sometimes to be totally driven by data is as wrong as to be totally driven without data" (May 1999). Managers from the former Beth Israel doubted the wisdom in relying on "data"—namely statistical measures—to the exclusion of qualitative experiences of patients and staff to modify practice.

In his speech to the BIDMC medical staff, Reinertsen emphasized that "the lopsidedness in managerial and leadership positions" contributed to "a lack of respect and understanding and acknowledgment and recognition of the unique ways of working that existed on both of our campuses," particularly those of the Deaconess. He validated the anger felt by the Deaconess staff, who felt that their potential contributions to the merged hospital had been too quickly dismissed and overlooked. He stated that this lack of recognition was "as big an insult as you can do, and it's painful, and it creates real victims."

During his speech, Reinertsen proceeded, in what many former Beth Israel employees regarded as a negative and unflattering account, to blame the current merger problems on the inadequacy of the Beth Israel management process. Reinertsen detailed the breakdown in decision-making brought on by reliance on the unwieldy Beth Israel management style, which "involved a lot of conversation. It depended enormously on the presence of a really remarkable individual, named Mitch Rabkin for it to work." He emphasized that without Rabkin around to "make that process work," BIDMC "developed no way of working."

Criticism from the new CEO, who had replaced the much-loved Rabkin was a hard pill for the Beth Israel folk to swallow. In 1998, Reinertsen replaced Mitchell Rabkin as director of CareGroup. Jonathan Cohn in an article in the *New Republic* described Reinertsen as Rabkin's diametric opposite. "Rabkin, an endocrinologist known for his human touch," the article stated, "personified Beth Israel's glory days." He urged collaboration among physicians and nurses, imbuing the hospital with an egalitarian ethic and "encouraged decision-making by consensus rather than dictate." This was in contrast to Reinertsen: "With his crisp business attire, aloof manner, and talk of hospital efficiency, he came across as more CEO than physician—exactly what the search committee wanted."[16]

Not only had Reinertsen acknowledged the Deaconess's power disadvantage in what was supposed to have been a merger of equals, but he blamed current merger problems on the inability of Beth Israel managers to lead without Rabkin. His praise for the Deaconess's achievements in TQM and the benefit of a data-driven system were perceived as a rejection of the relational style of the former Beth Israel leadership and a signal of changing values in the organization. Rather than placing a premium on relationships, the new leadership valued efficiency and measurement. These values would guide the hospital in its efforts to reinvent itself in the wake of not only a failed merger but escalating financial troubles.

Another Turnaround Plan

If the merger brought BIDMC to its knees, then the 1997 Balanced Budget Act, with its cuts to Medicare payments, hit the hospital while it was down. The BBA hurt all of the Boston-area teaching hospitals, but it hit BIDMC, which was already burdened with merger woes, especially hard. Early in 1999, the hospital estimated that its shortfall for the 1999 fiscal year would be close to $57 million, a deficit of over one million dollars a week. Reinertsen sounded the alert. BIDMC was in Code Green.

The hospital leadership decided that they needed outside consultants to help them. BIDMC hired the consulting firm Deloitte and Touche to assess the hospital's cost-cutting needs and "opportunities" for budget reduction and revenue increase. An administrator involved in engineering the turnaround plan described the relationship between BIDMC and the consultants: "We are the client and they are the pro. They have come in here because, for whatever reasons, we needed the will and the spine to do the things that in fact we knew we needed to do. The reason you bring in consultants is because you need that little nudge that you otherwise can't give yourself." The "nudge" came in the form of advice about areas where

[16] Jonathan Cohn, "Sick; Why America Is Losing Its Best Hospitals," *The New Republic,* 28 May 2001.

other hospitals or businesses managed to cut costs. According to the administrator, the consultants "do a comprehensive survey of what they call 'opportunity,' which is an interesting choice of words. An opportunity to cut costs or to increase revenue, both go together. . . . [They] serve up a menu, and then the organization itself reacts and responds. . . . So, together you kind of shape where you are going to go for revenue improvement and cost cutting" (June 1999).

In March, the hospital rolled out its plan for radical restructuring to cut costs and increase revenues—the keys to remaining viable in this new health care marketplace. They dubbed the resulting restructuring plan "Genesis." While the leadership had tried to give the program a name with biblical overtones and the sense of a new and important beginning, the medical and nursing staff jokingly but darkly renamed the program "genocide."

Genesis proposed a "core process redesign" aimed at capturing $90 million for the organization through a combination of "cost reduction and revenue enhancement," with particular focus on continued consolidation of the two hospitals. Projected cost reductions involved "approximately $23 million in labor costs from initiatives such as management and [General Medical Education] redesign, as well as reorganization efforts in lab consolidation, information services, pharmacy, nursing, and radiology" (internal memo to BIDMC leadership regarding Genesis Briefing Talking Points, 23 March 1999). It also involved restructuring of the administrative management team, a move that culminated in the elimination of eighty positions,[17] breaking from the former Beth Israel's no-layoff policy. This move also required a shifting of management duties and functions at the vice president level, which entailed the renaming and realignment of departments to reflect their functions in care delivery, rather than clinical disciplines.

While the clinical staff understood the hospital's need to restructure and cut its budget, they felt excluded from this process. For them, the hospital leadership's reliance on outside consultants signaled an emphasis on business values and a disregard for the medical expertise that used to guide

[17] "Beth Israel Deaconess Cuts 80 Management Positions," *Associated Press State and Local Wire,* 22 May 1999, Business News.

decisions. Many staff members felt that the hospital wasted money paying "big bucks" to "suits" who did not understand the intricacies of clinical practice. As a nurse manager explained: "This whole Genesis process is being designed by people who don't work in the trenches. . . . They think it's simple" (May 1999). An administrator described the common feelings of clinicians and others not directly involved in the redesign process "that somebody else, somebody out there, somebody up there who doesn't understand my work is making these decisions, and no one tells me anything, and no one communicates with me. . . . Where in the world did they come up with these ideas? And if only they understood my practice and what I do, I could fix it, but no one ever asks me" (June 1999). These feelings were all the more jarring because "everybody had the fantasy that it would be a redesign process." With the organization closely scrutinizing all of its practices from admissions to purchasing to resident training, employees on the front line expected that they would be tapped for their opinions and insights about how to make processes more efficient, cost-effective, and patient centered.

An administrator explained, "These design processes promised in people's heads that . . . people in the front line would say this is what works, this is what doesn't work, this is how you fix things. And I think, at least initially, that is not where things have started." For the most part, front-line employees' input was unsolicited; they did not participate in the task forces or meetings to decide the organization's future. The administrator explained, "When you look at the guest list, it is executive directory, physician organization—it is very high level. . . . It is a restructuring not a redesign."

Sharon O'Keefe, the new Chief Operating Officer and the woman driving many of the restructuring plans, had ambitious plans for change in the organization. She joined the BIDMC management team early in 1999, after having served as Senior Vice President of Patient Care Services and Operations at the University of Maryland Medical System and before that as a senior manager at the consulting firm of Ernst and Whinney. An administrator explained that O'Keefe envisioned a very different organization at the beginning of the next fiscal year: "When she says different, it's where [managers] manage to our budgets and [make sure] that people perform. I mean it is very performance based. It's a scary thought. You know, because your history doesn't matter a whole lot. It's how you perform, and it is a very business order. . . . O'Keefe's vision is that managers who manage will have enhanced accountability" (June 1999).

Genesis focused on realigning departments—putting items under jurisdiction of the appropriate manager and into the right budget. These changes focused on paperwork and billing and accountability, but not on how processes actually happened on the ground. At the same time, managers and employees were going to be evaluated based on how well these processes worked—based on performance. But many of the changes proposed by Genesis had very real consequences for performance—for the front line's ability to continue doing the work of the organization. Losing or gaining a new manager, coping with layoffs in one's department, moving to another department, or dealing with newly created or consolidated departments while also learning new systems and paperwork had ramifications for how work would be performed. Yet the potential obstacles and their implications for clinicians and patients had not been examined. No one outlined how patient care would actually be delivered on a daily basis.

In reaction, clinicians began to question the values of the organization and its future direction. Another administrator explained that the organization's current financial focus "lumped the nurses and physicians together more, all against the administration." She explained that the clinical staff had united around patient care concerns, "It seems to me like they're in the soup together" (March 1999).

Doctors and nurses alike expressed the feeling that the patient-centered values of the organization were taking a "back seat" to budget considerations. An administrator involved in the restructuring plans validated this viewpoint while also justifying the hospital's stance: "It's that cliché of no margin no mission. And that is kind of where we are. We've got to get to margin so we can get mission back again. . . . When an organization is really trying to right itself, that is the first order of business. I've had nurses say to me that . . . our values have gone out the window. I don't think that's true. I think that the current value right now is on survival. It's kind of a hierarchy of needs. . . . First things first" (June 1999).

The hospital was in dire financial trouble and needed to make significant financial gains before it could take the time required to thoughtfully redesign processes. If the organization could not resolve issues of margin, it would not be around to concern itself with mission, administrators said. This was the justification for the focus on finances. A physician described the situation and the need to change with the times: "We're all being put with a gun to our head, that if you continue to do things the way we did things, we are going to be a non-entity. . . . You can't lose a million dollars a week and survive. . . . And we're frustrated. . . . We don't get the time with the patients that we once got. . . . Its not a happy place for us. . . . But if you don't make the changes, you're going to be doing catering" (June 1999).

Despite the prevalence of this viewpoint among managers, many of the nurses I interviewed rejected this reasoning. If the hospital could not serve patients, then what was the point of its financial survival? How could mission be divorced from margin as the hospital pursued restructuring strategies? And what would happen to patients in the meantime while the hospital tried to respond to Code Green?

2

No Working Model for Nursing Practice

Before I officially began my research, one of BIDMC's board members confided that even though Beth Israel and the Deaconess had officially merged and were supposedly the same hospital, he still would much rather be admitted to the Beth Israel part of the medical center. Why? Because of what he felt was a striking difference in the quality of nursing at the two institutions. The Deaconess nursing service could not hold a candle to the professional, personalized nursing care provided at Beth Israel, he said. During a board meeting, he related his preference to Joyce Clifford, the head of nursing at the merged hospital and the driving force behind Beth Israel's prestigious nursing program. According to the board member, Clifford assured him the hospital leadership was working hard to implement Beth Israel–style nursing at the Deaconess. They would soon have the Deaconess nursing service "whipped into shape." Instead, within a couple short years, Clifford, all of her management team, many of her nurses, and her nursing model would be the ones who felt "whipped."

How could Clifford have been so wrong? The answer lies in an understanding not only of the different cultures of the two hospitals but also in the cultures of their nursing departments. Over the decades prior to the merger, the two hospitals had developed different nursing practices, and nurses worked from different conceptions of their role in patient care. Although Beth Israel strove to implement its professional nursing practice on the Deaconess campus, the culture around nursing at the Deaconess presented a formidable barrier to acceptance of Beth Israel's primary nursing model.

Changes at the whole institution posed an even greater obstacle to building and maintaining Beth Israel–style professional nursing practice on the two campuses. As the hospital restructured in response to its failing finances, nurses' work was unintentionally and haphazardly redesigned. Restructuring at the hospital introduced multiple changes in nurses' daily work, but little thought went into the effect of these changes on nursing practice. Restructuring undermined the elements that had made the different models of nursing practice successful on each campus prior to the merger and diminished nurses' ability to plan, implement, and evaluate care for their patients.

Different Nursing Models

Beth Israel nurses were convinced of the superiority of their nursing program and shared Clifford's confident assessment that Clifford would "whip" nursing at the Deaconess into shape. In 1995, just one year before its merger with the New England Deaconess Hospital, Beth Israel was featured in *The Best Hospitals in America: The Top-Rated Medical Facilities in the U.S. and Canada* (1995). The book specifically mentioned the quality of Beth Israel's nursing program and its achievements in building a professional nursing practice around the concept of primary-care nursing:

> If a hospital is to be judged on the quality of its nursing program, Beth Israel will certainly be rated one of the best in the country. Its nursing department has been cited as a model for nursing practice by the *New York Times,* the *Boston Globe,* and many professional journals. . . . Beth Israel was selected by the American Academy of Nursing as one of 41 magnet hospitals in the United States and was asked to participate in three national studies examining nursing care, which were sponsored by the Division of Nursing Health and Human Services, the National Commission on Nursing, and the Institute of Medicine. In addition, nurses from more than 20 countries and 20 states have requested either a field placement or observation experience at Beth Israel during the last five years . . .

> The primary-care nursing program at Beth Israel, developed in 1974, has one of the longest and most successful histories in the country and has served as a model for many other hospitals. Each patient is assigned a registered nurse, who is responsible for developing a coordinated individual care plan. The primary nurse accepts 24-hour accountability for maintaining continuity of care from admission to discharge or transfer and provides direct nursing care to primary patients and other assigned patients while on duty. This hospital-wide system allows nurses to give more personalized care and helps ensure that competent care is maintained throughout hospitalization. (Wright and Sunshine 1995:164–5)

Beth Israel had gained national and international recognition as a pioneer in developing and nurturing a professional practice model for nursing.

Beth Israel nurses were accustomed to a parade of visitors from other hospitals, not only from the United States but from all over the world. These guests came to learn about Beth Israel's primary nursing model. Beth Israel nurses, in addition, sought other outlets to publicize their achievements. They published widely and promoted their model in lectures and visits they made to other institutions around the world.

The Deaconess nursing service, although it had not received either the accolades or the publicity of Beth Israel, saw themselves as being on the cutting edge of practice of a different kind. In the early 1990s, the New England Deaconess Hospital became a pioneer in restructuring. Among the first to recognize trends in the industry, it introduced new, supposedly more efficient ways of providing patient care. To save money, the hospital downsized its registered nurse workforce and built a program of training patient care technicians to take over the less-skilled work traditionally performed by nurses. These tasks included bathing patients, changing bedpans, and taking vital signs. While other hospitals also made use of unlicensed assistants, the Deaconess program distinguished itself with an innovative, intensive three-month training program.

This program promised a clear definition of the assistant's role and mastery of the skills needed to perform it (Wiggins, Farias, and Miller 1990). The remaining nurses, with the assistance of the patient care technicians, were supposed to be able to manage a larger patient load comfortably. An administrator from the former Deaconess Hospital emphasized the benefits of this arrangement: "A practice assistant . . . can do many things that extend the hands of all care deliverers without affecting the process because it frees up the nurse and physician, who can do only certain things that no one else can do. So you take and you extend the hand so that they can do the high-level things they have been critically trained to do" (June 1999). Another administrator boasted, "for three years we reduced costs by 10 percent—the variable cost which is pretty significant. We did it by streamlining, taking out non–value-adding work" (July 1999).

Initially unhappy with these changes and worried for their future jobs and for patient care, the Deaconess nurses considered unionizing. During the 1993 union campaign by the Massachusetts Nurses Association, the union was defeated by a two-thirds margin. Hospital administrators attributed this substantial victory to the nursing leadership's efforts to communicate the benefits of the new program and its importance for the hospital's financial health. Consequently, the Deaconess nurses prided themselves on their ability to provide high-quality care with fewer resources. A representative of the Deaconess nursing leadership went so far as to claim: "Quality-wise, I'm sure you'd see no difference, and costs [at the Beth Israel] certainly were not less. When you take that balanced score card measurement, we overachieved what the BI did because we were sensitive to the cost, which they weren't. . . . We were sensitive to patients and what they wanted, not what nursing thought they needed. . . . [Nurses] felt good about what they were doing. . . . because they could see their contributions, but they could also see how they had to work with less" (July 1999). The Deaconess model emphasized nurses' dual missions as employees of a financially strapped hospital and as caregivers; it thus claimed to combine caring with cost-efficiency. The Deaconess nurses prided themselves on the care they delivered to patients and their active role in the hospital's financial performance.

However, the Deaconess nurses had trouble articulating the features that distinguished their nursing practice. They referred to it as "a way of working." When pressed, they pointed to the introduction of patient care technicians as a defining characteristic and innovation of their model. The Deaconess nurses and administrators continually claimed that they did the same things with patients as the Beth Israel nurses; they just did not try to do everything by themselves. They claimed that there were no real differences in daily practice, except that the Deaconess nurses had learned to be more efficient and could handle a larger patient volume.

The Deaconess rank and file seemed unaware of the extent to which their roles had actually been redesigned. The Deaconess Hospital had done more than just add some nurse-extenders. It had further parceled out nurses' role in patient care by adopting what was called "differentiated nursing practice." An article in *Nursing Management* by Judith Miller, the head of Deaconess nursing, and colleagues from the Deaconess outlined the changes to nursing that the Deaconess introduced in response to cost pressures in the late 1980s and early 1990s. The task force redesigning nurses' work at the Deaconess had "observed two different styles of practice. Some nurses preferred to deliver direct care to patients without assuming broader planning and coordinating responsibilities" (Harkness, Miller, and Hill 1992:27). The hospital created the position of clinical nurse (CN) for this type of nurse. "Other nurses," in contrast, "were more challenged by analyzing patient needs, evaluating patient progress, coordinating care for groups of patients and promoting cost-effective utilization of available resources." For these nurses desiring different challenges, the patient care manager (PCM) position was created. The patient care manager assumed twenty-four–hour accountability for planning, coordinating, and evaluating a patient's care—what the Deaconess designers referred to as the "primary nursing functions" (27). The PCMs would oversee the work of CNs, whose role, to use the language of primary nursing, was conceived as one of "associate nurse," to whom the primary nurse delegated particular patient-care tasks for her patients on a shift basis. While at Beth Israel any nurse could be a primary nurse or associate nurse at any given time, at the Deaconess these were fixed roles, corresponding to nurses' preferences and training.

The differentiated practice model at the Deaconess recognized that nurses' preference for a more active or passive role in patient care typically corresponded to their level of education and experience. Nurses could follow one of three different educational routes to become a registered nurse: four years of education at undergraduate institutions to earn the bachelor of science in nursing (BSN); two years of education at a junior college to earn an associate degree; or three years of hospital-based training leading to a diploma in nursing (Bednash 2000). Whatever the academic course, nurses completing any of these programs took a state exam to earn their registered nurse (RN) license (Bednash 2000).

When the Deaconess Hospital sought to redesign nurses' work, many of the hospital's nurses had earned their diploma in nursing from the Deaconess's own diploma school of nursing, which closed in 1989. Others earned associate degrees or diplomas in nursing from other nursing schools. Nurses with bachelor degrees in nursing were in the minority. All of these nurses were RNs, but, as in most other hospitals, they had "been assigned interchangeably in the workplace without regard to either their academic preparation or their experiential background" (Harkness, Miller, and Hill 1992:26). However, there were differences in the competencies of nurses graduating from four-year baccalaureate programs compared to the less prestigious associate degree and diploma programs. In particular, lesser-trained nurses were prepared to provide care to clients "who have common, well-defined nursing diagnoses." Moreover, this care needed to happen in "a structured health care setting . . . where the policies, procedures, and protocols for provision of health care are established" (Primm 1987:222). In contrast, a nurse with a BSN was competent to provide care to patients "with complex interactions of nursing diagnoses" in settings that "may not have established policies, procedures, and protocols and has the potential for variations requiring independent nursing decisions" (222).

In redesigning nurses' work during the nursing shortage of the late 1980s, the Deaconess chose not to recruit BSN–trained nurses. Rather, it chose to accommodate the comfort level and competencies of the majority of its nurses by creating a more routinized role for them. The hospital developed "critical pathways"— detailed protocols for providing care to the typical patient with a particular diagnosis. These critical pathways "could be used to monitor patient progress each day according to accepted norms" (Harkness, Miller, and Hill 1992:30). The critical pathways charted the patient's anticipated responses to treatment and acted as a standard of care, providing a basic recipe for the care the clinical nurse provided. Any deviation from the expected course would be brought to the attention of the physician and patient care manager, who would then reevaluate the care plan.

The Beth Israel nursing leadership looked down on the Deaconess's differentiated practice model as a deprofessionalization of nursing. The Deaconess hospital administration, by dividing tasks among patient care managers, clinical nurses, and patient care technicians, adopted the process described by Harry Braverman as increased division of labor. In this process, management separates work into its constituent elements and breaks it down among workers (Braverman [1974] 1988:52):

> Every step in the labor process is divorced, so far as possible, from special knowledge and training and reduced to simple labor. Meanwhile, the relatively few persons for whom special knowledge and training are reserved are freed so far as possible from the obligations of simple labor. In this way, a structure is given to all labor processes that at its extreme polarizes those whose time is infinitely valuable and those whose time is worth almost nothing. This might even be called the general law of the capitalist division of labor. (57–58).

This process resembled a reversion to the "team nursing" of the 1940s and 1950s. In *team nursing,* a skilled, registered nurse—regardless of which type of training program she had completed—oversaw inexperienced or less educated aides, who were responsible for direct patient care, while the nurse herself had limited contact with patients (Gordon 1997). Team nursing broke down the nurses' role in patient care into pieces that could be performed by workers with varying levels of skill. In so doing, it defined nursing practice not as a holistic process of providing care but as a series of tasks to be carried out. These tasks, many mundane, did not all seem to require the expertise and judgment of a professional nurse.

The primary nursing care model established at Beth Israel Hospital had been a response to and rejection of team nursing. Primary nursing sought to reintegrate care activities and return direct contact with patients and control over their care to a qualified nurse at the bedside (Brannon 1994). In its formulation, primary nursing elevated the professional status of nurses by defining even mundane tasks as part of a complicated process of evaluating patients, planning and implementing their nursing care, coordinating that care with other members of the care team, and continually reassessing the efficacy of interventions.

The development of primary nursing at Beth Israel was a long-term process of which the institution was enormously proud. A decade earlier, in the late 1970s, the Beth Israel nursing leadership had faced a dilemma similar to that faced by the Deaconess nursing leadership in redesigning nursing practice. Few of the nurses at Beth Israel had BSN degrees when the hospital introduced primary nursing. However, as Clifford explains in an essay about the development of Beth Israel's practice model, "the close relationship of the nurse with the patient promoted through the system of primary nursing called for an increase in the educational preparation of the staff." These relationships "call for increased communication, collaboration, and consultation in order to effectively coordinate care on a continuum. Nurses began to tell us in all kinds of ways that they simply were not prepared with the requisite skill and knowledge to meet the expectations they now held for themselves" (Clifford 1990:47). Rather than reduce expectations and roles, the hospital continued to demand more of its nurses, many of whom chose to return to school to gain the desired skills. To reduce the frequent turnover from nurses returning to school, Beth Israel adopted a hiring preference for BSN nurses.

The different paths the two hospitals took in designing nurses' role is reflected in the population of nurses working at the two hospitals at the time of the merger. The vast majority, 94 percent, of the nurses at Beth Israel had four years of education at undergraduate institutions to earn their BSN. Additionally, many were seeking or had already completed the two to three years of additional training to earn a Master of Science degree, usually in a specialized subfield. In contrast, only 43 percent of Deaconess nurses had attained the BSN degree.

Barriers to Extending Primary Nursing to the Deaconess

The Beth Israel leadership believed that differences in educational preparation contributed to differences in the culture of nursing at the two institutions. More educated and experienced nurses would be more assured of the value of their insights and judgments, more insistent on sharing these with their colleagues to promote the patients' best interest, and more eager to take an active role in planning a patient's care. Not only did Beth Israel select this type of nurse but the hospital also strove to create an environment that supported nurses' efforts to advocate for patients and take an independent role in planning nursing-specific care. The Beth Israel nursing leadership contrasted this with what they saw as the more passive, subordinate role of nurses at the former Deaconess, where the doctors "ruled the roost." They described the passive attitude of the Deaconess nurses: "We work for the doctors, and they tell us what to do, and we follow their orders" (April 1999). One nurse executive described the difference as follows: "On both campuses, nurses would question a physician's order if they thought it was wrong. On one campus they would question it, and doctors would say, 'No, that's what I meant.' And they said, 'OK.' On another campus, they'd question, and the doctor would say, 'No, that's what I meant.' And they'd say, 'Are you sure? Why are you doing that? That's not the right thing.' Push, push, push. Now which is right and which is wrong?" (March 1999). The Beth Israel nursing leadership thought that their way was right. They hoped to elevate the practice of all of the Deaconess nurses to the professional standards set at Beth Israel.

In the merger, the head of nursing at Beth Israel, Joyce Clifford, became the Senior Vice President of Nursing and Nurse-in-Chief. In an obvious snub, the former head of nursing at the Deaconess, Judith Miller, did not even receive a post in the new Nursing Department. Miller, the former President of the American Organization of Nurse Executives and a recognized leader in nursing in her own right, was instead installed in the Department of Patient Care Quality, where she had little input into nursing practice at BIDMC.

After the merger, the Beth Israel nursing leadership attempted to extend their professional practice model, and particularly primary nursing, to the Deaconess campus. The Deaconess nurses, who had been paid hourly wages, became salaried, and a number saw an increase in their pay. Additionally, the Deaconess nurses became eligible for professional advancement and promotion, and some took advantage of the program.

Despite these changes, the culture of nursing at the Deaconess provided a strong barrier to disseminating Beth Israel's professional practice model. At the time I arrived at BIDMC in 1999, nurses on the Deaconess campus claimed to be practicing primary nursing. The Deaconess nurses had grudgingly adopted the primary nursing method of patient care assignments, where the same nurse was assigned to the same patients throughout the course of their stay. Many of the Deaconess nurses complained that this was a step backward from the way of working they had utilized before the merger. The Deaconess nurses favored their old method of patient assignments, which assigned nurses to patients in neighboring rooms. Since patients might move rooms during their stays, this method did not ensure continuity of care. However, it conveniently concentrated a nurse's patients into the same geographical space on the unit rather than scattering her patient load across the unit. This arrangement reduced the time nurses wasted traveling back and forth across the unit to care for patients, and the close proximity of the nurse's patients made it easier to keep abreast of any changes in their conditions.

Although the Deaconess nurses had changed their method of patient care assignments, Beth Israel nurses insisted that this in itself did not make their practice true primary nursing. Although I myself witnessed no consistent differences in practice between nurses on the two campuses, Beth Israel veterans observed marked deviations from Beth Israel's professional practice. In particular, they noted the reluctance on the part of Deaconess nurses to do more than fill doctors' orders for patient care. The Deaconess nurses did not seem to take ownership of the nursing care their patients received, they said, but rather carried out the steps outlined in detailed standards of care and seldom deviated from the basic recipe. According to Beth Israel nurses, Deaconess nurses were competent in the care they delivered patients, but they did not take the extra step, fundamental in primary nursing, of assessing the adequacy of a treatment plan for a particular patient and of generating new solutions when a patient's response to treatment showed room for improvement.

Roberta Freidman,[1] a nurse who had spent her entire career at Beth Israel, was struck by the differences in culture between the two hospitals and how those impacted nurses' care plans. Freidman observed that the Deaconess reinforced the "division of nursing and physician" through symbolic practices, such as separate conference rooms and separate notebooks for nurses' notes and care plans, that emphasized nurses' position as subordinates rather than as colleagues. This contrasted with Beth Israel's emphasis on collegiality between nurses and physicians and the placement

[1] Interviewees' names have been changed.

of nurses' notes and care plans in the medical record alongside those of physicians and other health care professionals. Freidman complained, "We're all professionals. I would rather see a more collaborative relationship. . . . There is an expertise to nursing that can be offered to physicians. You try to offer as much as you can to the physician group about the patient and the care . . . But sometimes I feel that it's more of a one-way street—Physicians saying, 'Let's do this; let's do that; let's do that'" (January 1999). She saw this division playing out in the lack of independent decision making of the Deaconess nursing staff. In her view, the Deaconess nurses tended to be more passive, less proactive in making their own care plans: "The staff asks much more of physicians over [at the Deaconess]. Whereas, I think we would make more decisions independently over [at Beth Israel], just say, 'Okay, why don't we do this?' . . . [On the Deaconess campus], 'Oh no, you have to get a physician's order.' You have to get a physician's order for everything. That can be a bit frustrating at times" (January 1999). The Deaconess nursing staff waited for physicians' permission or approval before changing elements of the care plan, even those elements over which nurses had authority.

In a separate interview, Lynn Edison, a longtime Beth Israel nurse who had also been transferred to the Deaconess campus, shared similar sentiments. She acknowledged a large base of similarities in practice: "The majority of the care is the same. If you look at the nursing practice you find that . . . there is . . . a huge overlap . . . : they are all getting evaluated; they are all getting their medication; they are all getting their dressings changed if that is what's needed; they are all getting fed." Despite these similarities, differences in culture impacted the care patients received.

Edison noted striking differences in the evaluation of patients "and then what people choose to do about what they've found—whether you just let it be or whether you actively change the care plan." Edison gave a scenario that showed the difference in approach: "If the patient is calling for their pain medicine and it is not due for another hour and a half, you can either go in there and say, 'It is not due until seven o'clock. So I'll bring it in right at seven. Okay?' Or you can go in there and say, 'Tell me about the pain. When did you feel the medication started wearing off? Does moving make it worse?' And then you can go and call the doctor and say, 'You know what? This is an inadequate dosage of pain medication. I gave it an hour and a half ago, and it has already worn off. Why don't we try this?' That is a different way of doing things" (February 1999).

Edison explained that "the thought process is totally invisible" when it comes to acting out one scenario or another, and visitors, like myself, from one campus to another might not observe any differences in what nurses did with patients. However, she asserted, "If you don't take it on yourself to understand the patient's situation—what the patient's problems are—you won't develop a plan to do something about them. That as we go along we'll just do what the doctor's orders say to do but not really do the nursing care. . . . That makes your job easier, but the patient doesn't get the care" or the pain medication when needed, and the patient in her scenario would have experienced the difference.

Edison gave an example that emphasized the consequences of the more active role she took with patients. Edison had a patient who had arrived several days earlier with a severe psoriasis outbreak. The psoriasis was not the primary reason for the patient's hospitalization, and the patient had not received proper treatment for her skin condition. Few if any of the nurses on the unit had ever cared for patients with psoriasis before, and, according to Edison, "They made no effort to find out how to take care of them. There was no effort to find out where they could get the patient into a tub, if one is available. . . . They've got a skin care specialist that nobody consulted with." She conceded, "These are unusual types of patients for the hospital to have. . . . You don't get a lot of patients with psoriasis." However, in her eyes this did not excuse her Deaconess colleagues from making the effort to learn, especially when they had so many resources at their disposal: "We've got dermatology clinics; we've got a nurse practitioner over there [on the Deaconess campus]. We've got resources in the institution that could have helped them, but none of [the other nurses] utilized them." Edison exclaimed, "You know, I've heard more discussion of the flakes of dead skin on the carpet outside the patient's door than how you take care of this patient, how do you get this dead skin off of her."

Edison began a care plan with the patient that involved soaking the patient in an Aveeno (oatmeal) bath and applying ointments; "I got about ten pounds of dead skin off that woman. It was unbelievable! She looked different after she got appropriate skin care. [After] three days in a row; she's well on her way to healing."

Edison highlighted the difference in perceptions of the nurse's role that drove the difference in approach to the psoriasis patient. She contrasted her approach with those of a nurse who waited for the physician's orders:

> They're not planning care with goals in mind . . . And if it [the doctor's order] only says, "Aveeno to skin twice a day," then somebody is going to say, "Okay, well, I'll soak some towels in Aveeno, and I'll put them on the rungs [of the bed]." Well, that's not enough. You won't necessarily know it's not enough if you haven't taken care of that kind of patient before. You wouldn't necessarily know what it's supposed to look like when someone with psoriasis improves. But with a little care and a little inquisitiveness you figure it out. [If] you took care of the patient three days in a row, and the skin looks exactly the same, you might figure that you weren't getting very far.

The difference hinged on evaluating the patient's response to intervention. According to Edison, if there was no response—the skin did not look much better after a few days of treatment—then a nurse actively managing a patient's care plan would think, "Maybe you should talk to someone about it. Maybe you should speak to the dermatologist about it. They're in here . . . every day. Maybe you should call the nurse practitioner in the dermatology clinic. She's there five days a week, ten hours a day. But nobody does. . . . And I just find that very discouraging. And that is a very basic part of practice, and it's easy to change."

She linked proactive behavior to experience: "More experienced nurses are more likely to be willing to make that kind of decision because you have to have enough background, knowing what works and what doesn't work and to be able to think, 'What would I try next?'" She conceded, "I think you find nurses like that on both campuses." Edison highlighted a critical component of this kind of care—institutional encouragement. She held that more nurses at Beth Israel adopted this more active role in evaluating patients and modifying care plans because of the culture that supported this type of professional behavior. She concluded, "It is easier to be active . . . when you've had a lot of success being active in the past and when you feel like that's your job" (February 1999).

According to Edison, the Deaconess nurses on her new unit were afraid to move beyond basic nursing decision-making. They did not want to develop individual care plans for each patient, not because they did not have it in them to do so but because they had no support to do so:

> I think the idea of coming up individually with a plan for a patient seems very frightening to them. . . . I think what you are seeing is the fear that they would make the wrong decision. They don't have the confidence in their own professionalism and their own ability to plan care for their patients because they were never allowed to develop it and they were never allowed to make those decisions. And it was not physicians who prevented that from happening—it was nurses. They are looking for someone to tell them what to do. (February 1999)

To the Beth Israel nurses, the Deaconess nurses seemed not to want to give up the comfort of the standardized practice that their differentiated practice model had encouraged. The Deaconess nurses seemed not to worry whether the care they delivered was appropriate if it was specified in a standard, and they did not have to go through the additional steps of searching for information or consulting other nurses. The standards, then, saved time and provided a measure of safety for nurses concerned about their judgment calls.

Aware of Beth Israel opinions about the inferiority of their nursing, the Deaconess nurses I interviewed felt very much the underdogs and were quite defensive. On my first day of fieldwork, a disgruntled nurse from the Deaconess complained, "They think our nursing is crap." The Deaconess nurses were proud of nursing at their hospital. In interviews and informal conversations, nurses from the former Deaconess Hospital consistently maintained that they delivered the same quality of care as the Beth Israel nurses, but in a more cost-effective, efficient manner. They thought that they had much to offer to their merger partner in terms of updating their nursing model to meet the demands of the current health care market and that their achievements had been too quickly dismissed.

In particular, the nurse administrators from the Deaconess were proud that they had figured out how to handle the financial pressures the hospital faced and still provide excellent care. In contrast, according to a former Deaconess nurse manager, the Beth Israel nurse administrators "were not at all close to where we are . . . with budgets, with staffing schedules. We were very structured, disciplined, lean" (April 1999). A former Deaconess nurse administrator compared the Beth Israel nursing staff to spoiled children in their attitude toward cost-effective changes: "There was no incentive in BI nursing to be cost-effectively innovative. . . . I'm not saying anything about clinical quality of care; I'm just talking about practice techniques that take work out of what you're doing and are cheaper to do and stuff like that. There was like no incentive to even look at their practice" (March 1999).

The Deaconess nurses held that, unlike the Beth Israel model, their standard-based practice provided a realistic balance of the patients' and the hospital's interests given the changing health care market. They saw the potential to update the Beth Israel nursing model, which they characterized as "fat," "antiquated," and less effective in an era of larger patient loads and dwindling lengths of stay. They portrayed Beth Israel nurses as sheltered children not ready for the harsh economic realities facing them and emphasized that Beth Israel's nursing model was too resource intensive to survive. Nurses from the Deaconess felt that their "structured, disciplined, lean" way of working better anticipated frontline nurses' needs and constraints and enabled nurses to continue to provide excellent care in a harsher hospital marketplace. Moreover, they were reluctant to let go of this more efficient way of working.

In a conversation among a group of nurses on the Deaconess campus, a Deaconess nurse defended the predominant method of practice on her campus. "[On the Beth Israel campus,] [t]hey have a lot of autonomy. Here we have more structure." She went on the offensive, pointing to the pitfalls of having so much autonomy: "They have too much independence and can bend the rules. With everyone doing things their own way, there's too much room for error. With so many patients and such a heavy load, it would be too easy to make mistakes. Maybe if I only had three patients and could get to know them really well, it would be nice." Her comment reflected the notion shared by many of the Deaconess nurses that the Beth Israel nurses, prior to the merger, had had lighter patient loads that allowed them to spend more time with their patients. "But it's not like that over on the BI-side anymore," she said pointing to the increased patient load and to the fact that designing a unique care plan for each patient required more time and left more room for error in a fast-paced environment. She claimed, "They're getting used to the way we've always done things here" where there have been a lot of patients with high acuity. Her comments and the clucking approval of the other nurses present highlighted the obvious pride in Deaconess nursing and an underdog sense of superiority that they had operated with a leaner system (Fieldnotes, January 1999).

I asked Edison about these comments during our interview. She responded that there were standards for patient care at the Beth Israel, but these were much more flexible than those at the Deaconess; the Beth Israel clinical guidelines encouraged tailoring care to the individual needs of the patient. In another interview, Freidman, a Beth Israel nurse who had also been transferred to the Deaconess, observed, "Standards often meet the needs of staff but not always the needs of patients." In her daily work, it frustrated her that her new unit on the Deaconess campus was "much more policy and procedure driven than [the BI] campus, that things are very cut and dried. You do it this way, and that's the way it is." She appreciated the "greater flexibility of practice" that she enjoyed when working on the Beth Israel campus since "every patient brings some uniqueness of care that won't fit into a standard. . . . I think you need to have policies and procedures. But I do think there can be some leeway in them that meets everybody's needs." However, she acknowledged that "there's comfort" in having the more rigid standards:

> I think why people feel comfortable with standards, is we used to have more resources available to us. So if you ran into an issue and you weren't comfortable with it, you could always call on a resource person to help you work through something. There was enough staff on the floor. You could kind of gather together and kind of all work something out together. . . . Well, there isn't time any more. You run from the minute you get here until the minute you leave. And, at times, you never get to see another staff person because you're just so busy. And when you can't collaborate and talk about practice, the standards are comfortable because you know exactly what to do. (January 1999)

In the face of time and resource constraints that made it more difficult for nurses to get the support needed to individualize care, the standards provided a safety net. However, for Deaconess nurses this safety net was being threatened with the forced extension of primary nursing to their campus. The less confident Deaconess nurses were being asked to take on greater responsibility for planning and evaluating care. In some cases the nurses did not recognize the greater accountability and responsibility imposed by primary nursing because they failed to see the difference between the standard-based care they delivered and the tailored, personalized care delivered by a primary nurse. Other nurses from the Deaconess recognized the difference in demand, though perhaps not quality, inherent in the different models of nursing practice. However, many of these nurses thought adoption of primary nursing's greater autonomy and flexibility unwise. The additional expectations placed on the primary nurse made them uncomfortable, and it was extremely worrisome in light of changes in the hospital industry and at BIDMC. These Deaconess-trained nurses worried that the flexible, individualized practice being forced on them would push them past the limits of safety and prudence as patient loads increased and work sped up on the units.

These nurses recognized something that those attempting to redefine their role in patient care did not. The Beth Israel nursing leadership undertook to bring the Deaconess nurses' into the primary nursing fold at a time when resources that supported clinical decision making were being cut to save money. Under these circumstances, it would be difficult to build the professional culture and confidence enjoyed on the Beth Israel campus. In addition to this complication, cost-cutting measures at the hospital undermined the predictability and structure that had supported the Deaconess's differentiated practice and enabled the care standards to work so well. Now, the Deaconess nurses, who had yet to develop as primary nurses, lost the option of reverting to their old way of working. Moreover, these same changes in the hospital challenged the competency of even the most experienced Beth Israel nurses to provide professional nursing care. In the end, both sets of nurses were left without an effective way of working, and all of the nurses in this study began to worry about their ability to provide high-quality care to their patients.

Problems with Primary Nursing

Despite their initial self-confidence in the ability of their model to predominate, by 1999 Beth Israel nurses were worried about the survival of primary nursing. When the practice of primary nursing had been introduced at Beth Israel in the early 1970s, most patients stayed at the hospital for ten to fourteen days (March 1999). In contrast, in 1999 most patients stayed about thirty-six hours, about a day and a half (March 1999). The primary nurse might only see her patient for one shift before discharge, rather than over several shifts. This situation challenged the basic conceptualization of primary nursing as a "holistic" and "comprehensive approach to patient care" based on "a longitudinal relationship across the whole episode of the illness . . . from admission to discharge" (March 1999). The shortened length of stay posed a challenge to forming therapeutic relationships with patients.

Kathleen Curtis, a veteran Beth Israel nurse lamented the dramatic change in her practice. She contrasted care in 1999 with the care she could provide in the late 1980s and early 1990s when there were lighter patient loads and patients stayed in the hospital longer: "Now, we have more patients and they are sicker. They don't stay here as long. . . . It's much more fast paced. There isn't room for the personal care that they used to get. There isn't time to get to know your patients as people as much because you don't have a lot of chit-chat time anymore." Frowning, Curtis confided, "There isn't primary nursing anymore. . . . It's not the way that it was. You don't know them at the level that you used to know them." Nurses now faced such an increased workload that primary nursing "doesn't happen anymore. . . . We still take care of people . . . but it's not at the same level."

The distinguishing factor between primary nursing and the nursing now practiced on her floor, Curtis explained, was "how personal you are, how if you walk in they know your name right away. You are able to give a piece of yourself." She mourned, "There isn't time to give a piece of yourself anymore. . . . It's a one-way relationship now. It used to be give and take. You'd sit on the bed with a ninety-eight-year-old man and say, 'So what did you do to live this long. What's your secret?' I don't have time to do that anymore."

In the face of this lack of time, Curtis struggled to deliver the same level of personal care that she had in the heyday of primary nursing. She recounted a recent example of giving care that she considered primary nursing. One of her patients was told by his doctor that he had lung cancer. In the same breath, the man was told he would be released from the hospital that very evening because he wasn't acutely ill enough to stay in the hospital another day. Devastated by the diagnosis, the patient and his wife were overwhelmed at the prospect of such an early discharge. They shared their concerns with Curtis: "His wife was very angry, and that's when she told me. . . . He couldn't walk, nothing. They lived in a second-story apartment. . . . Just basic things. . . . She was completely out of her mind."

Curtis took it upon herself to make the extra effort that would help this patient and his family: "I did a little finagling. I called the attending to talk to him, to see what we could do." She then went a step further and "called the insurance representative herself, who was very defensive." Curtis managed to disarm the insurance representative by insisting, "Your role is to get them out, and I appreciate that. But my role is to protect them. So appreciate me, and we'll work together." Through Curtis's efforts, the patient stayed a few extra days. "He went in on Friday and he ended up staying until Monday . . . until everything was set up at home." The grateful family "cried. They thanked me. And I thought, 'This is why I do what I do—when you feel like you can make a difference if you just give them a little bit extra'" (March 1999).

Curtis's account points to the heart of primary nursing: the nurse's relationship to patients and their families. Taking the time to know the patient allowed the nurse to address issues of continuity of care that ensured that the patient receive appropriate services and support when he left the hospital. Curtis talked with the patient and his family to understand their unique needs, did the legwork required to get those needs met, and provided emotional comfort and support to the patient and his family. However, her efforts to involve the attending physician, to negotiate with the insurance representative, and to identify the patient's extraordinary needs at discharge (i.e., beyond medications and a referral for follow-up care) required a large chunk of time. With an increasing workload, such examples of personal care—of what the staff considered true "primary nursing"—were becoming fewer and farther between.

The problem was not just that patients' stays were shorter, but nurses also had less time to spend with patients on the days when patients were in the hospital. Journalist Suzanne Gordon, in her book *Life Support* (1997), describes the type of care that nurses at the old Beth Israel Hospital provided to patients in the years preceding the merger with the Deaconess. In several different accounts, she portrays nurses as spending a half hour or more talking with patients to help assess patients' needs, encourage patients' understanding of and willingness to follow a treatment regimen, or to provide comfort and support to patients or their families. In contrast, in the nine months that I shadowed nurses at BIDMC, I never once saw a nurse sit down and talk with her patients or their families—not even for five minutes, let alone half an hour.

BIDMC had clipped its average length of stay by almost half a day (0.4 days) since the merger, from 5.01 days in 1996 to 4.6 days in 1999. In reducing the number of days in the hospital, BIDMC, like hospitals across the country, cut out the part of the stay when patients, already on the road to recovery, required less hands-on care from staff. Stays were limited to the period when patients needed the most care and monitoring—the period when they needed the most time from nurses. Now, nurses did not have a mix of heavier and lighter patients; instead, they only had the heavy patients. Although on most of the inpatient units at BIDMC, the case mix—the severity and type of diagnoses—had changed little between 1997 and 2000, the needs of the patient population had increased. The rise of postacute care services in the health care industry meant that only the sickest patients required inpatient hospitalization. Together these trends filled hospital beds with more acutely ill patients during the time when they needed the most care. However, since the case mix had not changed, the hours of care that nurses were budgeted to spend with their patients did not change either.

While the average hours of care assigned to a case mix value did not change, the hours of care required to care for a caseload of patients with the same diagnoses changed significantly in nurses' experience. A nurse described the situation "Now nobody gets to stay to recuperate, so you don't have those lighter ones any more. The load is heavier, so it is more patients and sicker patients, so it's a challenge. So, I think people do find they can't do all the things they want to do, even some things that they know are very important. They don't have time to do it" (February 1999). Nurses were no longer able to average the greater hours of care needed by the "heavier" patients with the fewer hours required by their "healthier" patients. Nurses found that patients all seemed to need more care under these conditions. The result was that nurses did not have enough time to meet patients' needs.

Moreover, the time that nurses actually had available to provide direct care to patients was dwindling. The decreased length of stay compressed the amount of time between admission and discharge. Admitting and discharging patients were both time-consuming activities for the nursing staff. Patients required a large amount of immediate, up-front care to get settled and stabilized on admission. Admitting a new patient to an inpatient unit often took an hour or more. Discharge required a good deal of paperwork, and it also involved planning and arranging for care at home or in another facility. With the introduction of a new computer system in 1999 in preparation for the Y2K glitch, discharge paperwork and preparation began to demand three or more hours of a nurse's time.

The increased frequency of discharges and admissions decreased available time at the bedside. A nurse observed, "You're spending a lot more time really focusing on the two aspects of the stay, which is admitting some people and discharging them. And from the time they're admitted you're trying to get them discharged. . . . It seems like that is taking up a larger amount of time than it used to. So I think that takes away from the time of planning and implementing the day-to-day care for the patients on the unit" (July 1999). Admitting and discharge preparation, activities, and paperwork ate a sizeable chunk of an eight- or twelve-hour shift. Moreover, on any given day, nurses might be discharging their full patient load and admitting a new set of patients.

The quick cycle of admission and discharge necessitated getting information about patients as quickly as possible in order to plan their care while in the hospital and to arrange services for postdischarge. A nurse described the chaotic conditions on the floors that resulted from everyone's needing information at the same time, "[The units] are zoos. And it has only intensified with the acuity changes in the last ten years. The patients are so sick. It's just hard . . . with the amount of coming and going, and phone calls, and people involved in direct patient care that need access to the patients and the charts. Those nursing stations are like the floor on the stock exchange. You can't get a chart; you can't find the chart; you can't elbow your way to the phone. Even with a dozen computer terminals, it's hard to get charts. I think the nurses are very stressed, and I think the physicians are very stressed" (February 1999). Hospital staff required a high volume of information about patients, and they had little time to gather it or to communicate with the various other team members contributing to a patient's care.

Not only did the staff need to access information about patients' conditions and needs in a hurry, but so did the patients' families. In a focus group, a nurse spoke to the greater communication demands that the shorter stays placed on the staff: "Their families need more information. Like everyone wants to know something. . . . It's like more people coming at you from more angles, that need more information. Because they need it, because they don't have twelve days to figure it out" (focus group, August 1999).

Nurses needed to communicate important information to patients' families in a more compressed amount of time than in the past. With patients leaving the hospital so soon, they were often far from recovered from their illnesses or operations at the time of discharge. Families required even more support and information from the nurse than in the past in order to arrange for the patients' care needs on leaving the hospital and to learn about medications and warning signals. Families' increased need for education and emotional support competed with other care tasks for nurses' time and attention.

The pressing need to retrieve, assemble, and communicate pertinent information about patients quickly and to numerous parties demanded considerable time, much of which was spent at computer terminals or in conference rooms. That this time was not spent at the bedside providing hands-on care made nurses from both campuses feel they did not have enough time to care for patients and in particular to perform "very important" physical care tasks.

Lack of time at the bedside challenged nurses' efforts to maintain professional nursing practice at BIDMC. However, the Beth Israel nursing leadership became defensive when confronted with statements by nurses that "there isn't primary nursing anymore." In a number of interviews, nurse administrators insisted that primary nursing still happened regularly, albeit in a different form. They claimed that with the shortened length of stay, care delivery might look different, but the basic tenets of primary nursing—"continuity and accountability" (March 1999)—governed daily delivery of care to patients throughout the hospital. A nurse administrator asserted, "You can call it anything you want, but it's the issue of accountability per patient, providing continuity to the patient, and really coordinating their care. The difference really is that patients aren't here as long. But is the nurse still accountable for the care of the patient? Yes she is. . . . Is the nurse accountable for trying to preserve as much continuity for a patient as possible? Yes she is." The administrator conceded, "Maybe it's just played out in a different way," but she held firm to the notion that primary nursing still governed nurses' actions, "To say that primary nursing is gone and dead and that we're not doing it—I don't agree with that. You can call it anything you want to call it, but the tenets of it are the same—to do good patient care" (April 1999). The Beth Israel nursing leadership refused to concede that primary nursing, the cornerstone of Beth Israel's professional practice model, was "gone and dead." They saw the current challenge as one of learning to maintain the basic tenets of primary nursing under a new set of constraints. The set of constraints, however, seemed to keep growing.

As part of the Genesis turnaround plan, the hospital introduced yet another challenge to primary nursing. In an attempt to boost nurses' productivity, BIDMC sought to expand the nursing assistants' roles and increase the scope of tasks they performed. This move represented an undoing of the careful reintegration of nurses' tasks that had occurred with the introduction of primary nursing in the 1970s. The greater use of nursing assistants challenged the very foundations of primary nursing.

Nurses took exception to the notion that "high school graduates who have a six-week training course" could take care of patients as effectively as skilled registered nurses. Nurses in the Emergency Department, where the role of the practice assistants greatly expanded as part of restructuring, argued that quality of care would suffer if assistants were substituted for registered nurses. An Emergency Department nurse asserted, "Don't think patients are going to be safe because they're not." She elaborated, "You can hire technicians to do all kinds of things and they can do a perfectly fine job at it. But the patient's safety and well-being is most well-served with a professional care provider standing right there, who's educated and knows what they're doing" (June 1999). In a separate interview, a second nurse emphasized the same point: "Whenever you take an unskilled labor force like that and try to put them in a position of caring for people's lives, this could be you or your mother or your family member, there's going to be a lapse in the quality. There has to be, there absolutely has to be." Nurses resented the idea that nursing assistants might push them out of their prized position as the primary caregiver at the bedside. They questioned what might happen to the quality of patient care if nurses relinquished their hard-won role as direct caregivers.

Nursing assistants were not new to either campus. However, in the past, their roles had been strictly limited, and nurses had more time to supervise them, often working alongside them. With the Genesis restructuring plans, nursing assistants now often performed their delegated tasks independently. Moreover, nursing assistants were being asked to take on a wider array of nursing tasks. BIDMC did not, however, adopt the Deaconess's intensive three-month training program for patient care technicians, but instead relied on a six-week training course. The nursing assistants now being introduced did not have the same level of competence and shared expectations at the outset as the patient care technicians at the Deaconess. Consequently, there was great variation in the value of these workers as assistants to nurses. (This had been a chronic issue among nursing assistants at the former Beth Israel Hospital, but it was less problematic when nursing assistants played a more marginal role and nurses had more time.) Some of the nursing assistants were nursing students, highly prized for their eagerness and growing knowledge. But their presence fluctuated around school schedules and semester breaks. The remaining nursing assistants had little formal training, and their assistance could sometimes be more hindrance than help.

Nurses had a vast collection of "horror stories" about the incompetence or questionable character of particular nursing assistants. One nurse described an incident in which a nursing assistant was emptying urine from different patients' catheters into the same container: "The cross-contamination there is phenomenal. So each catheter she went to, to empty, she'd already emptied someone else's catheter into that container. In other words, there was nothing malicious. She just doesn't have the knowledge or the educational background to realize what an absolute infectious disease nightmare that is" (July 1999). On one of the floors that I studied, nurses repeatedly complained that their nursing assistants hid during their shifts to get out of doing work. They told me that they often found the assistants sleeping on the job. The nurses even lodged a formal complaint against a couple of the nursing assistants, whom they accused of coming to work high on more than one occasion (Fieldnotes, March 1999).

Such negative experiences made the nurses that much more appreciative of "good" nursing assistants, who could be invaluable on busy shifts. "Good" nursing assistants could be "very helpful" to nurses by taking on tasks that are "time consuming . . . when you have a critical patient or many critical patients," one nurse said, cataloguing some of the ways: "Taking people off of bedpans, answering call lights when you're tied up, . . . giving some TLC, helping them get their lunch, doing a blood pressure, maybe drawing that second blood culture that you need" (June 1999). Competent and proactive assistants, the majority of whom were nursing students, could do much to lighten a nurse's burden, and nurses often expressed gratitude for the nursing assistant who would change a messy bed, give a bath, or make a patient more comfortable without having been asked.

At the same time, nurses were keenly aware that they were ultimately responsible for the actions taken by nursing assistants. As the nurse observed, "When it comes down to it, it's my license that's at risk. . . . I'm the one who's going to be in trouble" (June 1999). The Massachusetts Board of Registration in Nursing, which issues registered nurse licenses to graduates of approved programs who have passed the national registered nurse examination, investigates and takes action on complaints filed with the board concerning licensed nurses' misconduct. In cases where nurses have violated a law or regulation or caused serious harm to patients, the board has the power to reprimand nurses, put them on probation, and suspend or even revoke their licenses. As managers of nursing assistants, nurses are responsible for ensuring that the assistant's actions comply with standards of safe nursing practice. Since nursing assistants are not licensed by the state, any misconduct or omissions on their part might result in dismissal from their position at the hospital. In contrast, the nurse overseeing the nursing assistant could face not only dismissal from her job but loss of her state license and, therefore, her ability to work as a nurse in Massachusetts.

Nurses felt uneasy about their increasing reliance on nursing assistants. They worried that they were "responsible for the patient" but "not able to be as on top of what's going on with the patient as we used to be" (May 1999). Increasingly, the nurses at BIDMC felt they did not have enough time with patients to assess their condition and recovery and to plan and implement their care. Even if someone else delivered the hands-on care, nurses needed time with patients to plan and assess what kind of care should be delivered—time which they did not have. At the same time, nurses remained accountable for the care delivered by these assistants. But they did not have time to supervise people whose skills, competence, and degree of motivation might be questionable—people who were carrying out care plans that nurses did not have time to construct.

The nursing leadership expressed sympathy for the growing discontent among nurses about their lost connection to patients, but they argued that the nurses needed to adjust their expectations given the new economic realities. As one nurse administrator asserted, "[Time with patients] is a big issue. A very big issue. Some of that I think is very legitimate, and some of it is really needing to learn how change. We just can't go back to before. . . . That's the loss that people are feeling. It's a loss that all clinicians are feeling. Nurses are in a very hard and unforgiving environment right now. . . . This is the environment that we are all trying to restructure for" (March 1999). Claiming that nurses merely needed to learn how to change ignored the sizeable obstacles that nurses now confronted in their daily practice.

Further Challenges to Daily Practice

To make matters worse, as part of restructuring, BIDMC downsized its medical program, closing two of the general medical units on the Beth Israel campus. As a result, many of the floors that had had surgical specialty patients, particularly units on the Deaconess campus, now received the overflow of medical patients from the emergency room. Attending to medical patients, who needed more complex and time-consuming care than surgical patients, disrupted the efficient practice of nurses on surgical specialty units. The standards and protocols that applied to the more predictable conditions of surgical patients might not pertain to medical patients, who often presented with complex or uncertain diagnoses and whose illnesses sometimes followed unpredictable courses. Nurses unaccustomed to working with this more challenging group of patients would be at a disadvantage in trying to plan their care. Nurses required more time and support to be able effectively to meet the needs of this new set of patients. But, with restructuring, time and support were in short supply.

Caring for medical rather than surgical patients increased nurses' workload. Edison explained that her surgical patients "may need a little light assistance to get to the chair, but then I can leave them there and they can call me if they need help. We are way ahead of the game compared to the type of medical patient that can be admitted to the hospital." She explained that the medical patients admitted from the emergency room "have to be on death's door" to be admitted. She described the typical types of medical patients: "Patients who are demented, patients who can't take care of themselves, who can't feed themselves, who can't talk, who can't walk unassisted. They can't do a thing for themselves" (February 1999).

Not only did medical patients require more overall care, but their care required more time and skill. According to Susan Lazarus, a veteran nurse on a surgical unit to which a number of medical patients were now being admitted, medical patients may require a lot of different medications: "They're on fifteen medications, four times a day. It takes a lot of time to get the medications together. And it takes a lot of time to figure out a way to get them into the patient, who doesn't feel well, who doesn't know who you are, who's not swallowing them." In contrast, most of her surgical patients had fewer medications if any: "So immediately you've got a couple of hours freed up. You don't have to do that." Additionally, the neurosurgical patients tended to have planned surgeries and came to the unit after the operations, while medical patients were fresh from the emergency room: "When [patients] come out of the OR [operating room], they've already had their admission assessment. . . . You don't have to go through the background assessment. When they come from the emergency room, you do. So it takes twice as long. So that's a lot of work." Lazarus asserted that with the greater influx of medical patients, "It's getting heavier on [my unit] now. Those patients are sicker; they're older; they're elderly; they're demented; they're incontinent."

Nurse Anne Dawson insisted that "the impact of that kind of change on the nursing staff . . . has been underestimated. . . . In cases like this, where there's just overflow of medicine, there hasn't been enough preparation of the staff. . . . It hasn't been acknowledged enough by management. And people get very stressed about that." She identified the source of the stress: "[Nurses] feel like they're not doing a good job. And many times, they're not. And they don't feel good about it." She specified that nurses are "doing an okay job, but they're not doing a great job" caring for overflow patients because of lack of expertise: "But there are nuances about certain practices that you learn only by time. Nurses learn things by seeing the same thing over and over again. So when you throw a zebra into a cage of monkeys, let's say, and you haven't ever seen one before, you can read the instruction manual on how to take care of a zebra. And you can follow the instructions. But the things that are unwritten or unspoken, that you would learn because you would have seen a few zebras behaving, are lost" (July 1999).

Dealing with the overflow of medical patients posed a challenge to nurses in terms of anticipating their patients' problems and needs. Nurses found it more difficult to develop care plans for patients with "different kinds of diagnoses than we usually see on a regular basis" because "you don't have any routine. So you can follow the specified orders, but you haven't had any chance to develop any expertise. So you can't even project any trajectory for the patients" (July 1999). Nurses inexperienced with certain diagnoses did not automatically know the best way to care for such patients and tended not to know what to expect or what signs to look for. Nurses on specialty units at BIDMC faced greater uncertainty when caring for the stray medical patient and felt less confident of their skills and judgment.

Nurses pointed to an additional obstacle involved in caring for the overflow of medical patients: The doctors caring for those patients were housed on a different unit in the hospital and unfamiliar to the nursing staff on other units. "That means that they're not around to ask questions and that they view it as a pain in the neck to come to another unit, basically," Dawson said, adding, "So it's difficult" because "part of the thing that makes a unit work and makes the flow work is if there's good communication between the house staff and the nursing staff" (July 1999).

Mary-Ann Ferguson, a nurse on the Vascular Unit explained that on her surgical unit on the Deaconess campus, "you get used to . . . dealing with five surgeons [so] that you know what they like [and] what they don't like. . . . Whereas when you get other types of patients—whether they're medical or other surgical services'—you don't know what the attending's likes and dislikes are. You don't know what the normal things are for a lot of these patients. And then you have to find out who's covering them, residents-wise" (March 1999). The house staff found themselves spread thin trying to tend to patients housed on several different units, and they often did not know the nurses caring for their patients—could not even identify them by sight. This made it difficult to share information, even as the nurses needed more information than usual to care for patients with problems that they did not usually see. Lazarus observed that her fellow nurses on the unit "are not going to be happy" about caring for more medical patients on a regular basis "because they don't have the support they would need to do a good job taking care of very difficult patients" (July 1999).

Compounding the problems of treating these new patient populations, nurses had fewer resources at their disposal to support their clinical judgment and skill development. Nurses no longer had the opportunity to consult their colleagues or specialists on the unit about the best method of treatment. "There used to be lots of unit teachers and people that we could call if you needed assistance," a nurse explained. "Now that's been dispersed. . . . It's no longer available. I think the nurses are being spread very thin and it's hard to do a good job—or the job that I felt like I was doing ten years ago" (March 1999).

Moreover, educational resources fell victim to the budget cuts. A nurse manager complained, "Resources, as far as staff education, completely dried up. There are no resources for staff education, as far as clinical specialists or things like that" (July 1999). Clinical nurse specialists had been an important educational resource for the frontline nursing staff. These nurse specialists did not have their own patient load; they guided staff through complex decisions and also lent a helping hand in difficult situations. In an attempt to cut costs, management eliminated or reduced the clinical nurse specialist position on many units. Not only did this decision remove a support for professional nursing practice, it also stripped units of an extra nurse who could be called on if the patient census surged during the day. Already spread thin, nurses could not easily turn to their colleagues on the unit for support and advice. In the survey of 147 nurses I conducted on six units, only 47 percent—less than half—said they had time to talk about patient problems with other nurses.

Nurse managers and frontline staff alike felt that the limited resources now available for staff development and education were inadequate for supporting clinical judgment and decision making. In-service workshops had gained popularity as an inexpensive way to train staff in new skills; nurses could go to a couple of hours of scheduled educational programming during their shifts to learn how to use new technology or treat a particular type of problem. However, nurse managers faulted in-service workshops as unrealistic solutions given the time demands on staff and the limited budget for staffing.

A veteran nurse, Lazarus pointed to the shortcomings of in-service learning for teaching complex skills. Nurses on her unit were being trained to read patients' cardiac rhythms so that the floor could accept more acute patients, who required more intensive monitoring. She complained, "It's okay if you've got a new piece of equipment that you just need to learn how to turn on and off and make it work. But it's no good if you have new equipment that you have to learn how to work with and analyze and use, like cardiac monitoring that we just had. . . . You don't learn to analyze rhythms from two days of workshops." She described the consequences of having inadequate ongoing training and support: "So, as a result, we've got a number of our patients on cardiac monitors, and the nurses don't know how to analyze those rhythms. . . . You know, it's a complex thing. . . . To me that's a very big problem."

She cited the example of a nurse on her unit who was concerned that her patient's readout showed pauses in his rhythm. Based on the readout, the nurse, who was inexperienced with using the new technology, thought that there was something seriously wrong with the patient—that his heart had stopped beating. In fact, the pauses in the readout resulted from an equipment glitch; the machine made an erroneous reading when the nursing staff turned the patient over in his bed. "We turned him over, and he had pauses," Lazarus explained. "The algorithm that runs this machinery was having trouble analyzing the rhythm [when we turned the patient over], but you can do better. Just because the machine says the patient has no heartbeat doesn't mean that the patient has no heartbeat."

"Believe me, if the patient is standing there, talking to you, they have a heartbeat. That's an equipment problem. And you don't learn that by going to an in-service. And this is an entire staff that has no experience. So who are they going to use as a resource?" (July 1999). This illustrates, she said, the importance of having ongoing professional development and particularly of having on-site clinical specialists to support nurses in their practice. Lazarus contrasted the "tremendous professional development," "wonderful mentorship experience," and "clinical nurse specialists to encourage and support their practice" that Beth Israel nurses had enjoyed in the past with the experience of new nurses of being "just kind of chucked out there and given eight patients—'Do the best you can, and nobody has time to talk to you, so don't ask any questions.'" As a result, she observed a "definite change" in practice: "We're not developing staff the way we used to. So I would not expect to be seeing the same outcomes. That doesn't mean that they'll never develop, but it's going to take a lot longer. And it's going to take a lot more to come from within the nurse. They need to do it themselves because we don't do it for them any more" (July 1999).

Other nurses shared Lazarus's concerns about the development of new staff, who did not have the benefit of mentoring and professional support. Dawson worried, "Having all new staff, just like buzzing around without any good role models, is a disaster because there's no way to learn except by your mistakes or by your experience. And then you're only learning . . . and you're getting better just based on your experience. But you'll never transcend to being great because you never saw greatness"(July 1999). Without professional development and support, less experienced or less educated nurses found it especially difficult to feel confident and in control of their practice, especially when faced with a new patient population and a shortage of time with patients.

A Sense of Crisis

Restructuring at BIDMC forced even the most organized and experienced nurses to rush around and to question whether they were delivering suitable care to their patients. The hospital's efforts at restructuring, particularly those undertaken as part of the Genesis plan, contributed to a growing sense of crisis among the nurses in my study. Before the hospital undertook its new turnaround plan, staff described the condition on their units as one of "controlled chaos" (Fieldnotes, February 1999). In contrast, by April, "frustrating" and "stressful" became commonplace descriptors of nurses' work conditions. The brisk clip with which nurses moved from task to task and room to room in January and February had become a full-fledged jog by September when I concluded my fieldwork.

In warning me about the brisk pace on a particular unit when I went to shadow nurses in early March, one of the nurses claimed proudly, "we boogie on this unit" (Fieldnotes, March 1999). But after the hospital increased its restructuring efforts, slam dancing might have been a better metaphor. Another nurse from the same unit gave a typical description of her work pace: "Now its all rush, rush, rush. I'm running all day long. Sometimes I barely have time to pass out the medications. And you work so hard, but the patients aren't satisfied. They only know how much you've been in their room, and it isn't much—maybe only a few minutes. And it's quick, quick, quick. I'm in and out" (June 1999).

Similarly, on another unit, one of the nurses that I followed during my fieldwork had been rather cheery though efficient with patients when I followed her in February. Although she had a load of very demanding patients, we had time to hear about their hospital experiences as the nurse engaged in the daily tasks of delivering medications and checking vital signs. When I visited the unit again in August, I walked into the nursing conference room to find the same nurse hunched guiltily over a sandwich. The call bells rang so continuously that they became background noise that could almost be tuned out. Although I had not even commented, the nurse apologized profusely for not answering the patients' calls immediately. She had not eaten anything all day, she said wearily. Seven hours into her shift, she felt like she would faint if she did not get something into her body. She scarfed down her sandwich and returned to the floor where she once again rushed from needy patient to needy patient (Fieldnotes, February and July, 1999). In an interview, a physician observed, "There are more and more stories coming from the floors about things that have gone wrong" (June 1999). He exclaimed, "If you go up on the floors, it looks like a large group of chickens that have no heads!" (June 1999).

By the end of my fieldwork, nurses such as Kathleen Curtis, Lynn Edison, and Roberta Freidman, who had worked hard to give patients "a little bit extra" and individualize their care, had turned their attention to the immediate problem of providing patients with the most basic of care. With all of the changes at the hospital, nurses were unable to use the practice models that had served them in the past. Not having enough information about a patient's conditions or individual needs made it difficult to plan care or to ascertain whether a treatment plan was working. Without the necessary educational resources, nurses remained unsure of the judgments they made with the little information they had. Finally, without enough time nurses could not actually deliver the care they determined their patients needed.

3

Dismantling Nursing

In March 1999, Joyce Clifford announced she was leaving the position of Senior Vice Président of Nursing and Nurse-in-Chief at BIDMC to become the Chief Nurse Executive at its parent company, CareGroup. She tried to put a positive spin on her decision. The move was a sort of promotion: Rather than guide nursing at one hospital, Clifford now had the opportunity to influence and build professional nursing practice at all of the hospitals in the CareGroup network.

A number of observers had a different take. They saw Clifford's move as a graceful, face-saving means of exit. They believed that Clifford did not really want to resign but could not deal with the current issues confronting her at BIDMC. She could not bear to deconstruct and redesign the professional practice model it had taken her and her team a quarter century to erect.

Whatever Clifford's motive, she did not anticipate the consequences of her departure from BIDMC. That departure opened the door for BIDMC's leadership to dismantle the powerful Nursing Department that she had built and to systematically strip nurses of their long-held influence in the hospital.

Nurses' Power at Beth Israel Hospital

When Beth Israel Hospital adopted primary nursing on its inpatient floors in the 1970s, the hospital also adopted a host of new organizational arrangements. The architects of Beth Israel's professional nursing practice argued that by meeting nurses' needs, the hospital simultaneously met those of patients. Beth Israel organized itself around nurses' work, supporting and encouraging the work that nurses did with patients.

One nurse administrator described the original thought process around organizational design at Beth Israel, "We're going to have these professional nurses concentrating on the patient's family and what's needed there. . . . What does this nurse need? What kind of supports does this nurse need? What kind of environmental change needs to happen?" (March 1999). Clifford, writing in 1990, explains that a prominent place for nurses in hospital management followed naturally from this orientation:

> Establishing an environment that supports professionalism requires the understanding and commitment of others, especially hospital administration. When nurses understand that they and the hospital share the same mission, that is, the delivery of quality patient care, then their commitment with the hospital to achieve the goals established by the organization takes on new meaning; the requests of each seem more reasonable and achievable. (31–32)

Clifford argues that nurses want to deliver quality patient care and to work in organizations that support them in this endeavor. To the extent that nurses believe they work in a hospital that shares this mission, they are willing to cooperate in pursuit of the organization's goals. Nurses, for example, would be more committed to a hospital's efforts to restructure and cut costs if they believe the hospital is dedicated to excellence in patient care. In order for nurses to feel that their interests are aligned with those of the hospital, Clifford says, nurses must have a hand in hospital management; nursing administration must be synonymous with hospital administration. Clifford explains, "Nursing administration and hospital administration at Beth Israel are not viewed as separate entities, but rather as unified management seeking a congruent goal—excellence in patient care" (32).

For two decades, the Beth Israel Hospital leadership followed this prescription for aligning nurses' and the hospital's goals. Clifford became a prominent member in the hospital management's inner circle. Rabkin, in an essay entitled "Ascent from Mediocrity: A Redefinition of Nursing" written for a volume on the history of professional nursing practice at Beth Israel, describes Clifford's central position in the hospital organization:

> From the start, Joyce Clifford has been a major member of hospital management in two respects—vice president of nursing—a top administrative role, with full involvement in the planning and management of the institution . . . and nurse-in-chief—a clinical chief as are the surgeon-in-chief, physician-in-chief, etc., attending the medical executive committee and other major sessions for information sharing, planning, and the making of overall institutional decisions on the delivery of care. Joyce Clifford is involved as a peer on both the administrative and clinical levels. (7)

Clifford's two titles ensured that nurses had a seat and a voice, which she raised consistently, at the organization's decision-making table. Moreover, the recognition of nursing as a clinical discipline in its own right promoted the recognition of floor nurses as professionals entitled to autonomy, authority, and control in their daily work. It also laid the foundation for a professional hierarchy in which nurses answered primarily to nurses, from the management of their units all the way to the office of the Vice President of Nursing. These organizational arrangements devolved a great deal of status and influence to nurses and concentrated substantial organizational power in the hands of the Nursing Department.

The nursing-only hierarchy provided the real foundation of the Nursing Department's power within the organization. The hierarchy encompassed all of the nurses working in the hospital. Regardless of where nurses worked in the hospital—inpatient or outpatient services, medical or surgical units, etc.—as members of the nursing profession they were automatically part of the Nursing Department and belonged to the Nursing Department's budget. Through this professional hierarchy, the Nursing Department retained control over rank-and-file nurses working throughout the hospital. Nurses reported directly to other nurses, not to nonclinical managers or representatives of another profession. Since nurses constituted the single largest group of care providers in the hospital and worked in almost every area, nursing's fingers extended into the workings of other departments. With such far-reaching budgetary control, nurses had the influence to shape other departments and services.

The unbroken reporting chain from floor nurses up to the chief nurse executive enabled nurse administrators to control the daily practice of bedside nurses. The nursing leadership attempted to direct nurses' practice through the norms of primary nursing, a practice model designed to enhance both patient care and nurses' satisfaction. Even after the merger, socialization into the primary nursing system remained so strong on the Beth Israel campus that even the newest of nurses could recite chapter and verse of the philosophy and had internalized the message that she was accountable for her patients' care. (See Chapter 2 for discussion of the primary nursing model.)

Nurse administrators perceived themselves as nurturing nurses' practice. While nurse managers had the authority to hire and fire nursing staff, Clifford (1990) describes their role as one of mentor rather than one of manager: "[The clinical nurse manager] facilitates the primary nurse's role by assuring that resources are available and provides the necessary support as clinical (primary) nurses learn the needed skills and competencies for their role and for continued professional development" (42). The control that nurse managers exert over nurses reporting to them was downplayed: "It is this position that . . . is most capable of assuring that standards are met and that an environment exists for nurse professionals to integrate their professional goals with those of the institution" (42). Similarly, one level up, the directors of nursing who report to the Vice President of Nursing, ensured "consistency . . . in the interpretation and implementation of the philosophy, standards, goals, and future direction of the nursing division" (44).

Nurse administrators at Beth Israel perceived their role as one of promoting professional nursing practice and supporting nurses' clinical decision making. The reporting chain imbued nurse administrators with the sense that they directly represented the interests of frontline nurses. They saw themselves as advocates for, rather than managers of, bedside nurses; they managed the care environment and the resources available to nurses, but not individual nurses.

There was a little bit of a fiction in all of this—the pervasive myth of the autonomy and independence of the nurses to shape their own practice. Nurse administrators managed frontline nurses' practice, however subtly and implicitly, through disseminating the primary nursing philosophy and then translating its implications for nurses' activities. Nurse administrators, moreover, were not the only parties, or even the most powerful parties, who had a hand in controlling nursing practice. The nurses' practice was shaped and constrained by doctors and hospital administrators as well. Even at Beth Israel, nurses were still fundamentally subordinate to doctors and administrators, although perhaps more elevated within the confines of their subordination than nurses at other hospitals. Not only did the nurse managers control nurses' practice through elaboration of the primary nursing model, but so did administrators and doctors by setting the boundaries of nurses' activities.

Through the organizational arrangements around primary nursing, the nursing profession retained a good deal of control over organizational policies and decisions and over nurses' daily work. The nursing leadership believed strongly in the philosophy that had led to the creation of these arrangements. The nurse administrators I interviewed consistently presented these arrangements of nursing representation and power as promoting the hospital's mission of patient-centered care. A nurse administrator explained: "I think most all of us realize that the nurses are the frontline person with the patient. If you're not representing the interests of nursing, then you're fundamentally not going to be supporting patient care in a great way" (February 1999). As a result, nurse administrators recognized "a huge need to make sure that nursing interests are always on the front burner." The nursing leadership felt that they simultaneously represented the interests of the nursing profession, rank-and-file nurses, patients, and the hospital. Moreover, given the organizational arrangements established to promote primary nursing, they viewed these interests as synonymous.

Distance between the Nursing Administration and Bedside Nurses

With restructuring, the interests that the nurse administrators considered to be equivalent and the values that they claimed to represent began to conflict as the focus of the hospital changed from quality patient care to institutional survival. BIDMC was losing over a million dollars a week in the 1999 fiscal year. Such extreme losses required dramatic action. New leadership was in place. It was unclear whether the values that guided the former Beth Israel, particularly the pride of place given nursing, would still be maintained. Nurses' relationships with patients had become less central as the hospital leadership's focus became financial survival and cost-effectiveness. Nurse administrators found themselves in a precarious position.

Most of the nursing leadership had built their careers developing and refining professional practice at Beth Israel in an era flush with money. They stood to watch their achievements crumble as changes at BIDMC rocked the foundations of primary nursing. Not only was their legacy in jeopardy, but so were their jobs. In fact, the ranks of the directors of nursing and the vice presidents of nursing had already been thinned with cuts in hospital management, and nurse administrators wondered who would be next. Difficult budget decisions had to be made. The nursing leadership defined their role as one of protecting the core resources that supported professional practice, particularly primary nursing. While the hospital struggled to regain its financial footing, they remained invested in preserving professional nursing practice—even if it was less expedient or comfortable for bedside nurses—because they viewed professional practice as the backbone of high-quality patient care. Indeed, it was through primary nursing that they had implemented such impressive standards of care quality.

At the same time, the nursing leadership recognized the strain that nurses faced as various supports—educational programs, clinical specialists, and support services—were sacrificed to save money. However, they believed bedside nurses exaggerated the immediacy of the situation. The nursing leadership expressed sympathy for bedside nurses' situation, but saw it as a sign of the times and felt powerless to change it. They looked to nurses to adjust their practice to the new environment and minimized nurses' complaints about problems with care.

For example, one nurse administrator observed, "The pace is different as far as . . . discharges and people not being in the bed for a long time. The nurses are busy. We don't have much down time, that's for sure." At the same time, she defended, "I don't think staffing has ever been better than it is now. I really don't." Not concerned by the faster pace, she identified "staff expectations" as the problem: "But . . . staff expectations are different. So you never feel like you're really in control. I don't think people feel like they're in control as much as they did before" (July 1999).

Another nurse administrator, although concerned about the nurses' perceptions, also expressed the view that nurses needed to change the way they performed their work: "We have fewer and fewer resources. . . . And it worries me significantly that we've whittled away at the bedside and that nurses feel somewhat unable to deliver the care that they would like to give." However, she did not identify nurses' inability to "deliver the care that they would like to give" as an immediate threat to patients. She observed that perhaps "nurses did things that they might not need to be doing and could be done well by another group." "Instead of doing everything for the patient" as they had under primary nursing, nurses need to give up some aspects of care delivery and focus instead on "the critical essential things that the professional nurse brings to the patient in the planning and coordination of care." The same administrator stated, "I don't think care is bad. I think we've done what we've needed to do, and I think clinicians work really hard. But I'd be worried if we whittled away any further from clinical staff. I'd be very worried" (April 1999).

The nurse administrators did not immediately grasp the seriousness of the situation on the floors. They recognized that changes on the units, such as the greater use of nursing assistants, required an adjustment to primary nursing practice. They did not, however, understand that primary nursing practice was being undermined, not modified, by these changes. As a result of changes, the model was failing nurses, who now found it difficult to know what they should be doing for their patients or how to do it with the available resources.

Why this discrepancy? Because restructuring had broken down the connection between management and clinical practice that existed at the old Beth Israel, the supportive, guiding role that nurse administrators had designed for themselves had begun to break down. Rather than spending their time on the floors with nurses, nurse managers shuttled from one meeting to another to discuss restructuring, particularly standardization of nursing practice across the two campuses and preparation for ongoing consolidation. With attrition and reorganization of units, some of the nurse managers had been asked to expand their range of supervisory responsibilities to include other units so that a nurse manager for one unit might now be responsible for two or even three units. This further divided their attention. Their presence on the units had been greatly reduced, and they were not available to mentor nurses struggling with daily decisions.

The directors of nursing confronted similar issues. Since 1990, when Clifford described the model at Beth Israel, their numbers had dwindled from six to two. Furthermore, the remaining directors had even greater responsibilities because they now managed units on both the Beth Israel and the Deaconess campuses. These directors had only just begun to develop relationships with the nurse managers under their supervision, and the staff nurses often did not even know to whom their nurse manager reported.

Not surprisingly, nurses felt out of touch with nurse administrators, who were preoccupied with other matters and brushed aside nurses' concerns about their work conditions and care quality. A nurse emphasized the distance between her and the nursing leaders in the hospital, "I think a lot of the nurses who are in an upper echelon, who are nursing bosses or administration, it's been so long since they've done floor nursing that I really don't think they have an idea what it's like to be down in the trenches" (February 1999).

The survey I conducted on six inpatient units during the summer of 1999 provided a disturbing picture of conditions "down in the trenches." Only 25 percent of the 147 nurses responding to the survey felt that they had adequate support services that allowed them to spend time with patients. Only 32 percent agreed that there were enough registered nurses on staff to provide quality patient care. Even fewer, 29 percent of the nurses in the sample, agreed that there was enough staff to get work done, and 57 percent claimed that they worked understaffed on a weekly basis, with 19 percent identifying understaffing as a daily problem. A full 78 percent of nurses complained of rushing to meet their patient care responsibilities on a weekly or more frequent basis, with 35 percent indicating that they rushed to meet their patient care responsibilities every day. A third of the nurses responding to my survey indicated that care on their units was less than good overall. They labeled the care as either "adequate," "poor," or "very poor." "It goes nonstop," a nurse stated, "That's hard. It's very hard.

It's frustrating because you feel like you're not giving the best care that people deserve all the time—what I feel like I should be able to give to somebody . . . , what I want to be able to do for a patient. But I don't feel like I am able to do that as well as I did before" (July 1999). In another interview, a distressed nurse anguished, "The care is shoddy. It doesn't feel safe, from a practitioner's standpoint. This isn't how I care for people; so I don't want to do this. I'm going to get nailed" (June 1999).

Nurses complained that their work conditions forced them to provide what they considered to be "shoddy" care, or inconsistent and sloppy care that failed to meet their quality standards and, most important, put patients at risk. Nurses worried about getting "nailed" should something happen to one of their patients. In such a situation, the individual nurse would be blamed and could possibly have her registered nurse license revoked.

Nurses faulted the administration for its unresponsiveness to what nurses deemed conditions that placed them and their patients at risk. In an interview, an exasperated floor nurse complained, "With staffing the way it is, with money being an issue, they realize our problems but there is nothing they can do about it. You get, 'Well, that's the way it is now' and 'that's not a priority right now.' Well, what is a priority? Being told that we need to do the bare minimum for patients now is unacceptable for me because what's the bare minimum for a patient?" For bedside nurses, there was a fine line between delivering the bare minimum of care and unsafe care. As one nurse expressed it, "They are getting the best care that we can physically give them. I'm doing all that I can, but I'm not as thorough as I used to be, and I'm afraid that things could be missed" (March 1999). While most of the time nurses interviewed felt able to deliver good care, all pointed to recent instances when they felt "scared" or that the care was "unsafe."

Despite the pervasiveness of this situation, nurses found the administration reluctant to make any changes that might help them. "Administration wants to . . . say, 'well, show us the numbers, show us why you need more support staff." A nurse bemoaned, "They don't just magically give it to us because we asked for it. . . . It didn't matter how loud we cried to administration, 'Listen. On a daily basis there are unsafe practices going on in this department.' . . . Unfortunately, there needs to be a negative outcome for them to say, 'Oh, okay.'" (July 1999). Here was the paradox of prevention. It was the nurses' responsibility to prevent the negative outcomes that might prove to administrators that resources were inadequate. Adequate resources, nurses insisted, should be made available to create good outcomes, not suddenly appear because a patient died.

It was not until several months into the study that the nurse administrators at BIDMC gained a clearer understanding of the crisis in care that floor nurses confronted. After data came back to them from the floors—increasing numbers of complaints from nurses and patients, the research I shared, and the stories and concerns raised by focus groups conducted by the Nursing Department with floor nurses on different shifts and both campuses—they sought to take action. But by then, they no longer had a seat of power in the organization.

Mistaken Assumptions

Hospital administrators, for their part, also questioned whether nurses exaggerated patient-care problems on their units. One upper-level executive acknowledged, "people are stressed at the unit. . . . There is clearly work that needs to be done." But this executive questioned the relationship between nurses' concerns about deteriorating quality of patient care and their budget decisions.

In the face of cost-cutting, the Nursing Department had to eliminate some positions to meet its new budget. This executive, who was involved in tightening the budget, felt that staff nurse positions should be protected and that budget cuts should come in the form of reductions in the "number of folks in the central nursing office." However, this was not the cost-cutting proposal that the nurse administration submitted. "What came back was a decision within the nursing structure to preserve the entire central nursing office and take resources out from the units—their decision." The executive viewed this decision as "unacceptable" because "this is not lining up with where I think the values need to be." "[Nursing] exists," he said, "to advance the goals and objectives of the organization and not solely to advance the goals and objectives of the professional discipline" (August 1999). To him, the nursing administration's decision to protect the central nursing office came "at the expense of direct care providers." The nurses were complaining about conditions on their units, but, he said, the nurse administrators were acting to protect the central nursing office. Why the inconsistency? he asked. To him, this was proof that bedside nurses' stated concerns about patient care were not shared by the nurse administrators. He felt the decision demonstrated greater concern for preserving the "central nursing resources [that] are advancing the profession of nursing" than for care at the bedside: "I have a big disconnect in my mind about why I hear a value for the patient care, etc., [but] I don't see it played out in terms of resource allocation. . . . So it is a big disconnect for me in terms of how the language lines up with the actions" (August 1999).

To nurse administrators, the "disconnect" did not, as the executive assumed, reflect their greater allegiance to the goals and objectives of the nursing discipline. They assumed that these goals and objectives coincided with the hospital's mission to provide high-quality patient care. This apparent disconnect represented not a divergence in goals but in priorities. Both nurses and nurse administrators shared a deep concern for the quality of patient care. Frontline nurses, however, focused their attention on the daily, short-term priorities of caring for their patients. Nurse administrators concerned themselves with the long-term priorities of preserving the professional resources that promote and enable high-quality nursing care. While the nursing leadership did not at first realize the full nature of problems on the units, they understood that changes at the hospital threatened nurses' professional practice and, consequently, the quality of care. In response, they struggled to maintain the professional infrastructure that had supported high-quality care for patients in the past and that they believed was the key to maintaining this quality in the future.

The problem here is endemic to restructuring efforts that take managers away from the staff they manage. Had the nursing leadership more quickly appreciated the many obstacles that bedside nurses faced, it is unclear how they would have chosen to allocate resources. Either way, budget constraints would have forced them to choose whether to sacrifice care quality now or later. While keeping available resources at the bedside would have served nurses' and patients' interests at the moment, eliminating resources that supported nurses' skill development and judgment would have severely compromised BIDMC's ability to maintain care quality in the future.

However, administrators outside the Nursing Department misinterpreted the perceived "disconnect" between bedside nurses' words and the nursing leadership's action as a clue to the "true" motivation behind nurses' complaints about problems with patient care. Rather than viewing the decision as a no-win choice between preserving care quality in the present or in the future, they saw an either-or decision of advancing the nursing discipline's interests or of promoting patient care. The hospital administrators mistakenly assumed that the nursing leadership's efforts to preserve professional resources related more to preserving the power of the nursing discipline in the hospital than to preserving the quality of patient care. Based on this assumption, hospital administrators dismissed bedside nurses' claims about deteriorating quality of care as representing professional self-interest rather than warnings about real threats to patient safety.

This construction of the problem created a vicious downward spiral. Hospital administrators had little patience for nurses' gloomy predictions about patient care when they thought these merely represented a ploy to protect or even to promote nurses' status and influence. As a result, they easily dismissed nurses' concerns as unacceptable resistance to change, motivated by a desire to maintain nursing's power in the hospital. They recognized that changes at BIDMC threatened the central role nurses played in patient care under primary nursing. They interpreted nurses' criticisms of declining patient care as a ploy used to reclaim the professional status they were in danger of losing with current changes.

One administrator, for example, labeled nurses' concerns "mourning" "around the loss of the primacy of primary nursing." From this viewpoint, nurses resented the fact that greater utilization of nursing assistants was displacing them from the bedside. The administrator conceded, "I do think that the nurses have a valid point. To look at the care of a patient solely in terms of the tasks that you do with that patient probably misses a lot. I do think that we are involved in a lot of that. . . . [But] the bottom line is . . . people are going to have to deal with it" (May 1999). While she acknowledged nurses were unhappy with the changes in their role in patient care, this change, she said, had little bearing on the quality of care that patients received: "It's relevant to the nurse. It's not relevant to the patient." (May 1999). The administrator viewed nurses' expressed concerns not as reflections of the quality of care patients received but as a resistance to fragmentation of their role and direct control over patient care.

Similarly, another administrator admitted that nurses were "pushed toward being mere functionaries" and that "the inner value added, your soulfulness, your clinical judgment, your capacity to be a real asset . . . all of that becomes less important." The administrator saw nurses' complaints as reflecting that loss, but attributed nurses' protests to "bitterness" about changes rather than to any true threat to care quality: "That takes out in your own personal experience, especially those who practiced over time, it takes out what you probably value as part of your practice. . . . Part of the bitterness here, quite frankly, has to do with the aging workforce who remember . . . the good old days" (June 1999). In this person's estimation, nurses' vocal concerns about care quality pertained to longing for the "good old days" and an inability to accept "other sources of gratification." These constructions of the problem delegitimized and downplayed its seriousness.

Hospital administrators assumed that primary nursing provided the basis of nurses' power in the institution but was only marginally related to the quality of care patients received. After all, they reasoned, other models like the differentiated practice model used at the Deaconess also enabled nurses to provide high-quality care and did not require that nurses exercise so much influence in the organization.

The hospital leadership did not recognize how the nursing leadership's attempt to preserve primary nursing, and with it nurses' direct control over patient care, affected patients. They disregarded the decades of studies demonstrating primary nursing's worth as a method for providing excellent patient care. They, instead, reconstituted primary nursing as a means of professional satisfaction for nurses and as a way to enhance nurses' status and influence in the organization. What administrators did not realize, however, was that primary nursing also provided the basic orientation from which nurses understood their role as professional care providers and from which they planned and delivered care. Hospital administrators thus did not recognize primary nursing as a critical component to quality care.

Nursing as an Obstacle to Restructuring

At the former Beth Israel Hospital, under Rabkin's leadership, the qualitative relationship between nurses and patients was at the heart of decisions about how to organize services and departments. Personalized nursing care had been the hospital's crown jewel, the basis for its reputation as the best hospital in Boston. In the leaner postmerger environment, nurses' relationships with patients were no longer automatically accepted and recognized as the cornerstone of quality.

The problem was exacerbated by nurses' failure to describe their contributions using the quantitative descriptions and data that carried weight with the new hospital leadership. An administrator observed, "When the economics hit and the questions started to be asked, 'What does a nurse bring to a patient?' they [the nurses] were ready with all these touchy-feely, unmeasurable types of things. Those things are all good and all important, but that's not what is driving the boat any more" (May 1999). In the harsher economic climate, the new hospital leadership dismissed the same contributions that had directed organizational structure under Rabkin and Clifford as "touchy-feely" and "unmeasurable." With financial concerns "driving the boat," the hospital wanted to maximize tangible contributions that could be measured and assigned a monetary value. Consequently, what nurses described as qualitative contributions to patient care were devalued and the rationale for nurses' central position in the organization questioned.

Nursing's power in the organization came to be viewed as an impediment rather than as an asset. One administrator characterized nurses as feeling that they have to control every aspect of the hospital and "pointing to everything else as being the reason why something doesn't work for me." "There's absolutely nothing acceptable about not having supplies, linen, transport all of those things available," the administrator explained, "but the nursing structure also needs to allow those departments to develop and design those services . . . as opposed to telling that [department], 'Here's what I want the jobs to be and roles and everything.'"

According to the administrator, there were support personnel available to "assume the responsibility" for various tasks, and the problem was "the nursing staff not wanting to let go." He viewed nurses as too concerned with protecting their professional turf to make things work and asserted with exasperation: "If we are providing this resource to do this work, allow them to do the work! And don't create this kind of combat zone over who is doing what and then treat those people as though they are incom-

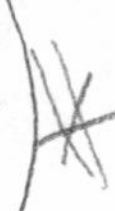

petent and unable to execute those duties." Although nursing had been "one of the strengths" of the former Beth Israel, the administrator explained that "people's sense of being able to work with the nursing structure is not one of being collaborative." He explained that "because of its size and presence" throughout different departments in the hospital, it was "the single biggest silo that exists in the organization" (August 1999).

One administrator described the Nursing Department as a "prima donna" in the organization (March 1999). Another administrator emphasized this same point: "When nursing in this institution was the power in the institution, they abused that power. . . . They didn't leverage their power in an inclusive way. They felt they could only operationalize that power by stepping on other departments, by bullying other departments" (May 1999). These comments reflected the view, shared by many of the administrators leading restructuring, that the Nursing Department had become self-serving, unwilling to be a team player in the hospital's efforts to restructure and to control costs.

Viewing nurses' protests over changes to care as self-promotion and resistance to change, rather than as patient advocacy, created a picture of nurses as obstructions to the hospital's turnaround attempt. The new leadership at the hospital insisted it was time for dramatic changes. Management at BIDMC moved to gain greater control over nursing in order to realign nursing's professional project and the hospital's struggle for financial survival. With the need to control costs, they argued, the "uncollaborative" Nursing Department needed to be reined in. As the hospital struggled with its finances, nursing—a powerful presence at the old Beth Israel Hospital—became a prime target for restructuring.

Demolishing the Nursing Structure

To gain greater control over nursing, BIDMC management dismantled the nursing hierarchy in which nurses answered only to nurses. The opportunity came in March 1999, when Joyce Clifford, Senior Vice President of Nursing and Nurse-in-Chief at BIDMC, moved up to the parent company, CareGroup.

Clifford either did not know or was in denial about what her transition would mean for nursing's status and influence in the hospital. She had handpicked her successor, M. Patricia Gibbons. Gibbons was regarded by many as Clifford's protégé. She had been part of the leadership team at Beth Israel from 1974 until 1982 and had implemented primary nursing at the unit level. She returned to BIDMC in 1998 as a Vice President of Nursing, after holding high-level nursing leadership positions in other institutions, including Vice President for Nursing at Yale–New Haven Hospital and Chairperson of the Department of Nursing at New England Medical Center. Clifford thought she was leaving nursing in capable hands.

The spring/summer 1999 issue of *Report,* BIDMC's newsletter on professional nursing, described the meeting of the nursing leadership group in which Clifford formally announced her transition to CareGroup and handed leadership of the Nursing Department over to Gibbons: "During the meeting, Dr. Clifford ceremoniously transferred the leadership to Gibbons by handing her the prized Adelaide Nutting Award [named for Mary Adelaide Nutting, who was Superintendent of Nursing at Johns Hopkins and credited with being the first professor of nursing in the world]. . . . Entrusting Gibbons with the safekeeping of the legacy, Clifford spoke fondly of the excellent leadership that her longtime friend and colleague brings to this new role."[1]

Although Clifford entrusted Gibbons with leadership of BIDMC's professional nursing program, the hospital undermined Gibbons's nursing leadership role. It rendered her powerless to protect or even to represent nursing's interest.

As part of the Genesis restructuring plan, Gibbons received a new title, Vice President of Patient Care Services, rather than being named Vice President of Nursing. Diluting her time and frequently her energy, she oversaw not the Nursing Department but a newly created department that included nursing as well as other professional disciplines, such as pharmacy, occupational therapy, and physical therapy. Gibbons's new title signaled that there was no longer an official Nursing Department; nurses were now part of the Patient Care Services Department. Inclusion in the department

[1] "M. Patricia Gibbons, DNSc, RN, Appointed Vice President for Patient Care Services," *Report* 3(1): 15 (1999).

did not depend on professional discipline but on delivery of inpatient care services, so the three hundred nurses who did not work on inpatient units, those in the Emergency Department and those in Ambulatory Services, came under the jurisdiction of those other departments. This move broke the reporting chain in which nurses reported to other nurses. Now, nurses answered to nonnurse and even nonclinical managers in the departments where they worked.

Despite Gibbons's protests, she was at first denied the title Nurse-in-Chief (although this situation changed a few months later). Removing this title signified that the hospital did not recognize her as the head of the nursing discipline. Most important, since no one else was granted the nurse-in-chief title, this move signified that the hospital no longer regarded nursing as a clinical discipline on par with other disciplines such as medicine and surgery.

A nurse administrator succinctly explained the changes: "Joyce was gone for twenty-four hours, and the other nurses were taken out of this department and reorganized into other sections. So the VP for Nursing and Nurse-in-Chief went to CareGroup, and a VP for Patient Care Services came in, and the organization was realigned, and all nurses did not report in to nursing" (April 1999).

Changes in the reporting structure opened discussions about issues related to other aspects of nurses' professional dominance. An administrator observed, "[Discussions] about where can nurses work in the organization, who can hire folks, what's their credentials—I mean each of those become personal assaults on the nursing structure" (August 1999).

Hospital administrators were fully aware of the symbolic meaning of the changes to the Nursing Department. A top executive outlined the significance of the titular changes:

> That means at the VP level the person needs to be imaged and viewed by their colleagues as being a key member of executive management and not the chief nursing officer. That sets the tone for the director level, for the manager level, and for the staff nurse level that really says that all things that are impacting the organization are opportunities for the nursing structure to help the organization position itself in the marketplace and to contribute to the overall goals. That is a huge change because this

structure had distinguished itself by advancing the profession of nursing and not necessarily being aligned with . . . the overall goals of the organization. (August 1999)

Hospital management demolished the nursing structure with the clear intent of weakening the power of nurses in the organization. The changes had their intended effect. A nurse administrator described nursing as "invisible, reasonably powerless within the organizational structure right now" (April 1990). By dismantling the Nursing Department, the hospital leadership severely reduced the control—over hospital decision making and over nursing practice—that nurses had gained in the twenty-five plus years of primary nursing. It was little comfort that Sharon O'Keefe, the new Chief Operating Officer who had orchestrated these changes, was herself a nurse.

This systematic assault on the nursing structure continued past the end of my fieldwork. The hospital summarily fired Gibbons in September 2000 and ousted the remainder of the Beth Israel nursing leadership by February 2001. The vice presidents, directors, and many of the nurse managers and nurses from the former Beth Israel Hospital left.

Nurses' Loss of Voice

Only one year prior to these changes, Clifford had authored a book entitled, *Restructuring: The Impact of Hospital Organization on Nursing Leadership*. She had conducted three case studies of hospitals undergoing restructuring and the changes to the nursing leadership's role in the hospital. Her book warned of the negative effects restructuring might have on nursing's ability to promote patients' interests. She documented instances of dismantling of nursing structures, of nursing losing its representation at the executive level, and of the Chief Nursing Officer (CNO) attaining responsibility for departments like Patient Care Services that included nursing along with other support services.

The irony in this is palpable. Clifford, perhaps naively, never expected restructuring to lead to such changes in her own hospital. One nurse manager observed, "a couple of months ago, Joyce spoke at a Seminars for Nursing dinner, and she talked about her experience going across the country, and how . . . the VP for nursing had been eliminated [at many hospitals]. . . . I'm sure she never suspected that that would happen here. . . . We've fallen so far and so fast" (May 1999).

Clifford, with her tremendous experience as a nurse leader and a research study behind her observations, expressed salient concerns about restructuring-related changes to nursing leadership in any hospital. However, as far as I could tell, BIDMC leadership did not share Clifford's concerns about the potentially deleterious and destabilizing effects of nurses' loss of powerful representation at BIDMC. In fact, the leadership seemed to dismiss such concerns. Nevertheless, in the BIDMC case, Clifford's warnings are prophetic.

In changing Gibbons's responsibilities, Clifford's own organization did not heed her warning that "distancing of the CNO's leadership role away from the professional domain of clinical nursing may ultimately have deleterious effects on nursing practice and, subsequently, patient care" (Clifford 1998:120). Similarly, when the hospital stripped nursing of its representation at the executive level, it ignored Clifford's observation from other hospitals:

> [T]he change in organizational identity has caused concern among nurse managers and other nursing leaders who fear the loss of their discipline's voice at the senior level of management. These concerns are similar to those voiced by nurses during the two national nursing shortages of the 1980s. During that time, clinical nursing staff felt their concerns about the delivery of patient care services were not understood at the highest level of the organization. They wanted to ensure that the interests of the direct care provider were understood and included in the organization's decision-making process. (106–7)

Clifford linked the current trends in restructuring to those during the nursing shortages of the 1980s. In identifying nurses' lack of representation as the common thread between those shortages and the current period of change, she implied that current restructuring could lead to a nursing shortage if nurses did not feel like they were active participants in the organization's decisions about patient care.

Clifford's study also examined the consequences for nursing leadership when hospital management dismantled the nursing structure, as they had done at BIDMC. She warns that this dismantling may have a destabilizing effect on the workforce and on the quality of patient care:

> The cohesiveness and infrastructure long associated with a central leadership and management structure for nursing services have provided stability, particularly as a communication vehicle, for the work of nurses as well as other clinical and hospital groups. As this structure is dismantled organizational chaos and workforce instability are major risks. One of the cataclysmic worries about breaking up the nursing department is the potential loss of an infrastructure that traditionally has provided a safety net for all of patient care. Those designing new organizational paradigms must consider these aspects of the structure, which for the most part have been taken for granted in the organization. (121)

Indeed, BIDMC took for granted the aspects of the nursing structure that provided a vehicle for presenting concerns about patient care and, therefore, a "safety net" for care quality. When BIDMC management took a wrecking ball to the carefully designed nursing structure, it did not set up a new structure to meet this need.

In making decisions about redesigning the nursing structure, hospital administrators considered changes at an administrative level. They hoped that by weakening nursing's influence, they would remove an obstacle to rapid decision making and change. Dismantling the nursing structure, they believed, would make the hospital a more flexible organization, better prepared to take action to control costs and increase revenues. The effects of these structural changes on frontline nurses and their ability to care for patients did not, as far as I could discern, enter into the decision. As a nurse administrator noted, "This is really what's happening in health care across the country. I think it's driven by the economics first and foremost. It's not always that they've carefully considered nursing and so have decided to put it there. It's that they're really being driven by the almighty dollar. So if you need to create this in order to maximize revenue and get patients in here as a business, then that's what you do. You don't worry about all this professional stuff" (April 1999). But "all this professional stuff" is important to the work that nurses do on behalf of patients.

In the hospital's economic crunch, nurses felt that "patient care is off the radar screen" because it did not generate revenue: "The primary worries here are market share, economics. . . . So there's been a tremendous shift" (April 1999). One nurse administrator related the powerlessness and invisibility of nursing to the loss of a patient-centered focus in the organization: "Whether its nurses or patients that you describe, it's off the radar screen. You won't find one without the other. You won't find a powerful Nursing Department that doesn't have a really patient-centered focus. If patient care is not a major priority in the organization, neither will nursing be. . . . We are a group that is sort of qualitatively responsive to the needs of patients. . . . I think it will swing back, but not until quality emerges as important again" (April 1990). This view that the fate of patient care was intimately tied to nursing's status position in the organization was widely shared by rank-and-file nurses. Nurses felt at odds with a hospital management that simultaneously chipped away at the nursing structure and at resources at the bedside.

Nurses experienced increased alienation from hospital administration and growing conflict between their role in patient care and the hospital's restructuring plans. With nursing's loss of power in the organization, nurses sensed that their interests were not represented in decisions about how to cut the budget. The hospital administration, they felt, was not adequately addressing their concerns about patient care and safety. The vast majority of the nurses responding to my survey, 76 percent, disagreed with the statement that the administration listens and responds to employee concerns. A nurse expressed nurses' shared sense of exclusion from organizational decision making, "I think we're doing more with less staff and people are unhappier. . . . I think a lot of decisions have been made with less input from the staff, less consideration of its effect on the staff." This failure to attend to the effects on staff led her to conclude that "patient care has taken a back seat" to other concerns (May 1999). Another nurse voiced the feeling shared by many: "I think there's a very clear message that there is no respect for nursing. . . . I don't have any trust in the administration of the hospital right now to do the right thing because I think they're too focused on cutting costs" (July 1999).

Nurses throughout the hospital felt a collective loss of control over hospital policies as the discipline lost its power and influence in the organization. Even those nurses unaware of the new hospital politics became painfully cognizant of the loss of respect and the relative powerlessness of their managerial "advocates." As resources and support dwindled at the bedside and frontline nurses' jobs became more stressful and difficult, nurses felt powerless to change organizational policies or to provide the care they thought their patients needed.

4

Power Contests and Other Obstacles to Providing Patient Care

On a typical day in the Emergency Department in 1999, patients waited. And waited. And waited. When they first arrived, they waited to be examined by the triage nurse. Then they waited for an examination room. Then for emergency room doctors and nurses to examine them. After that, they waited for tests, lab results, consultations, and assessments from doctors from other departments.

Once the ED staff stabilized an incoming patient, their ability to provide further treatment could be hampered by delays or problems with any one of these tasks. A backlog in radiology could mean an additional two-hour wait for a patient to be x-rayed and for the results necessary for diagnosis to be delivered to the ED team. Problems with updating, entering, or retrieving information in the new computer system could make the diagnosis and treatment process more cumbersome and time-consuming. The slowdown in caring for one patient often had a ripple effect, creating longer and longer waits for the next patients in the queue.

Within the cramped ED, space was at a premium. Waiting patients, who had already been admitted to the ED, occupied space needed for other patients. With frequent bottlenecks, only the most urgent emergencies would be treated, while other slightly less sick or suffering patients anxiously remained in the waiting area. Patients being admitted to an inpatient floor also waited to be transferred. Patients who had been stabilized and were awaiting transfer might be wheeled on stiff hospital gurneys into the busy ED hallway, where they enjoyed neither quiet nor privacy.

On one particularly busy day, a patient, a workman who had fallen from a ladder onto an iron rail, arrived to the ED in great pain with, staff suspected, several broken ribs. The triage nurse had to send him to the registration and waiting area because the ED beds were full and he was still moving and conscious (Fieldnotes, June 1999). While in terrible pain, he had to wait for several hours on the stiff benches in the waiting room. The scene was reminiscent of *ER* or the work conditions more prevalent at an underfunded public hospital, not what one would expect in one of the best hospitals in Boston.

Nina Harris, a nurse who had worked in the Beth Israel ED for over fifteen years, explained that these delays were not trivial for patients: "Patients wait, mostly. And they get miserable while they're waiting. They hate to wait. And we're not talking waiting 20 minutes, we're talking waiting four hours, waiting five hours. They wait for a million hours for things that, if we were a smooth-running machine, wouldn't happen." Harris pointed to the process of admitting patients to the Deaconess campus, a few blocks away from the ED, as a major source of delays:

> Transferring patients to the other campus is a nightmare. . . . We transfer lots of them over there. . . . And it feels wrong to have somebody come in by ambulance, to care for them, to admit them to our own hospital, and put them in an ambulance and send them down the street to be readmitted once again to another place. You just feel awful that you're doing this to people. So the people who get admitted to the other campus have much more delays than the people who go upstairs here. (June 1999)

The process of transferring a patient from the Beth Israel campus emergency room to an inpatient bed across the street regularly added an hour and a half to a patient's stay in the ED. The ED staff had to arrange for an ambulance to move the patient. Since the hospital did not have its own dedicated ambulance for transporting patients internally, staff needed to call an ambulance from the community. To add to these problems, protocol prohibited the paramedics from moving patients with intravenous (IV) lines. A doctor had to accompany them, or the IV lines had to be removed and reconnected when patients arrived at their destination across the street.

Problems with admitting patients accounted for the majority of hours logged waiting. The Admitting Department had to find a vacancy for the patient on an appropriate unit, move the patient there, and arrange for the receiving department to be ready for the patient's arrival. Problems at any point in this process meant that patients had to wait in the ED, even though they had already been treated, before they could be transferred to a more comfortable setting.

The need to coordinate admissions across two physically distinct campuses added to the time and difficulties involved in admitting patients from the ED. Since the consolidation of the Admitting Departments onto the Deaconess campus, in a plan officially called "Project Bedlam" (a name reflecting the dark humor and low morale even at the highest levels in the organization), the process had become bogged down. The aim of the project was to enable staff to create a clearer picture of the vacancies on the two campuses so that patient assignments would take best advantage of areas with available beds and staff. Management was working to create trust in the process, but perceived an "uphill battle" (Fieldnotes, March 1999).

Before the merger, at the former Deaconess Hospital, a "bed meeting" which took place every morning had facilitated this planning. A representative from each unit reported on the anticipated discharges, admissions, and staffing resources. While these meetings continued regularly on the Deaconess campus, the newly merged Admitting Department struggled to institute the same daily meeting on the Beth Israel campus. Resistance on the part of the Beth Israel nurse managers and difficulty in the ability to predict discharges due to differences in the patient populations (the medical patients on the Beth Israel campus had less predictable patterns than the surgical population on the Deaconess campus) prevented these meetings from being as fruitful.

In the meetings I observed, Beth Israel nurse managers or representatives attended the meetings with insufficient information on patient discharges. Even when they had the necessary information, they hesitated to disclose potential vacancies if they thought they did not have sufficient staffing to take more patients. Unwillingness or inability to communicate pertinent information made it difficult to keep track of vacancies and slowed the process of matching patients to units. In the meantime, the ensuing scramble to find beds for emergency patients delayed care and contributed to the stress for ED staff and patients alike.

Demand by referring and attending physicians that their patients be sent to one particular campus compounded the logistical inconveniences of coordinating care across the two campuses. Physicians affiliated with the merged hospital often held strong preferences for one of the premerger hospitals. Their identification with the premerger hospitals, and in some cases merger-related resentments or loyalties to colleagues they felt had been badly treated during the merger process, led to a lack of acceptance of the medical center as a unified entity. Their demands threatened the tenuous coordination and collaboration across campuses. As a doctor in the ED complained in an interview,

> And it's still not a merger. I still have to fight with doctors on the East [Beth Israel] Campus when I have to send their patients to the West [Deaconess] Campus because there are no East Campus beds. If you are one institution, you have to be able to cross the street and forget where your office is for a second. And it's one thing if your office is in the East Campus and your patients are at the West Campus. But when your office is [three miles away] in Jamaica Plain and you give a damn about which campus your patients go to, that's not a merger. Now you're just pissing people off. (June 1999)

Such demands from physicians, if met, could delay care while patients waited for a bed to open. If unmet, these often petty demands led to lengthy argument with the physician on the other end and served to increase frustration for an already busy ED staff.

A Breakdown in Coordination and Cooperation

In 1999, BIDMC had just begun to tackle the challenge of coordinating care across two distinct facilities. While the two former hospitals attempted to function as one, they had not, in the hospital staff's opinion, consolidated enough to make coordination across the campuses a simple matter.

The difficulty coordinating care across the two campuses profoundly affected nurses in the ED. The Beth Israel and Deaconess emergency departments merged in October 1997. This was the first clinical department to consolidate and now served both campuses from its location on the Beth Israel campus. The ED escaped most of the hardships involved in bringing together rival staffs from the two hospitals because there were relatively few Deaconess employees working in the merged department. Most of the physicians in the Deaconess ED were moonlighters, employed full-time at Beth Israel. Therefore, few Deaconess physicians had merged into the ED. Additionally, most of the Deaconess ED nurses took severance packages, and only a handful joined the new department.

Despite this, the ED faced a number of restructuring-related problems because it coordinated its operations across both of the campuses and depended on processes in other departments to function smoothly. Glitches or breakdowns in systems or operations in the hospital profoundly affected processes in the ED, which, though located at the former Beth Israel, served both campuses. Diane Nelson, a nurse in the ED, explained:

> [The ED] is an intolerable place for people to work. There are broken systems at every single bed. Everything that you have to do to take care of a patient is confounded by breaks in the system. We have issues of our own, I have no doubt. But we are also victimized by a dysfunctional organization. . . . The Emergency Department doesn't exist in isolation. We are totally dependent on the systems, all systems throughout the hospital. Whether they are information systems, laboratory systems, radiology systems, house staff systems—we are totally dependent on all of those. We don't exist on our own, and we're pushing against them every step of the way. (May 1999)

While restructuring-related frustrations registered greater effect in the ED than in many other departments, the daily frustrations faced by the ED nursing staff nonetheless provide insight into the effects of restructuring on frontline nurses throughout the hospital. Like ED nurses, nurses throughout BIDMC felt increasingly powerless to overcome the multiple system breakdowns and other obstacles that interfered with care delivery.

Due to merger-related resentment and disappointments, employees at BIDMC had become territorial and protective of their domains. One administrator described the deterioration in "basic collaboration and shared expectations" accompanied by the attitude "'I have what I want, I'm gonna get what I want, blah, blah, blah, and hell with the ramifications or how anybody else wants to do it.'" To illustrate how this new territoriality—even around some of the simplest activities—could compromise patient care and raise the blood pressure of the staff, she recounted the following incident. The manager found a dumpster that needed to be emptied on a daily basis and that was not being cleaned out. To arrange for daily emptying, she assigned the job to her staff. She was not sure who would end up paying for the garbage pick-up, but that was not, to her, the relevant issue. The main concern was that a garbage dumpster needed to be emptied every day; let's get it done.

What should have been a straightforward request to a colleague, turned into a convoluted exercise in detective work, when her staff reported back to her that the person who was responsible for paying to empty the dumpster had refused to authorize payment and thus garbage removal. When she set out to discover who this recalcitrant administrator was, she discovered he was a colleague with whom she had worked closely at one of the former premerger hospitals. She called him to discuss the problem, and he apologized for his failure to authorize payment with the excuse that "I didn't know who asked" for the garbage to be removed. The administrator exclaimed, "It shouldn't matter who asked. The thing's full; it needs to be emptied. Gimme a break!" (March 1999).

Employees at BIDMC reported that this type of behavior made it increasingly difficult for them to do their jobs. The lack of teamwork that informants and I observed throughout the hospital obstructed efforts to solve problems or bypass systems that were not working.

An administrator explained the importance of the shared history among coworkers: "Even back before the merger, even when you were mad at somebody, or you thought somebody was doing a lousy job, you'd known them forever. It was sort of like the sibling thing always tempered everything you did" (April 1999). In the more hostile, uncooperative postmerger environment, not knowing the person on the other end could be a detriment because there were no long-term relationships to temper the current power disputes.

As the hospital greatly expanded with the merger, departments consolidated and contact people changed. In comparison with both premerger hospitals' historic rates of low turnover, BIDMC suffered high turnover after the merger. In the Nursing Department, human resource records[1] showed turnover at a rate of 20 percent in fiscal year 1998 and 19 percent in fiscal year 1999, when it had only been 2 to 3 percent a year in either hospital before the merger. Turnover was thought to be even higher in nonclinical departments.

For hospitals that had enjoyed relatively little turnover, these developments were not only unprecedented but disruptive. Employees frequently did not know their peers in other departments. The shifting around of personnel through hospital growth and turnover meant that many people were new to their positions and also needed time to become proficient working in their new roles and with systems that were sometimes new both to them and to the hospital.

Merger-related hostilities only added to inefficiencies, as employees harboring bitter feelings were less willing to cooperate or find solutions when things went wrong. The informal routes staff had taken to settle disputes between departments or to fix system breakdowns became dead ends. This was particularly unfortunate because such problems cropped up more frequently due to integration of systems, introduction of new systems, and employees' inexperience in their new positions or resistance to new arrangements. Formal changes in the organization highlighted the gaps in the fabric of the informal social networks among employees as these gaps hindered implementation of restructuring initiatives. They contributed, furthermore, to employees' stress. Hospital employees struggled to overcome the difficulties of managing and adjusting to changes while performing their usual duties without the customary support and cooperation. They nostalgically remembered feeling part of a "family" and treating one another with respect, a sense that was heightened as the impersonal and sometimes territorial postmerger interactions among departments decreased cooperation, increased dissatisfaction, and made frontline staff, particularly nurses, feel a growing sense of powerlessness to overcome these obstacles and perform their work.

[1] For a time after the merger, BIDMC was unable to consolidate its human resource records. The first available data on turnover across both campuses are from 1 January 1997, and I only have this data for the Nursing Department.

A Heightened Workload

For the ED staff, negotiating their way through these roadblocks and delays in patient care added to an already heightened workload. Two years earlier, in 1997, the hospital had consolidated the two emergency departments into one location on the East Campus. Soon after, the volume of patients in the new ED exploded. Harris described the situation, "I think that we were as busy as you could possibly imagine, and then they added eight thousand or ten thousand patients, however many [the Deaconess] used to see a year, to our workload without accommodating them" by adding new staff or providing greater space. Despite the widely held perception that the increased volume resulted from absorbing the eight- to ten thousand Deaconess emergency visits along with the sixty thousand to seventy thousand that Beth Israel saw yearly, hospital administration insisted that the increased volume was actually the result of having a broader physician referral base from affiliation with the CareGroup network. Whatever the cause of the increased volume, nurses in the ED felt that the hospital failed to make appropriate adjustments for the greater workload.

"I think they turned their back on it and said, 'Oh, make it work, do the best you can,'" Harris explained, echoing the widely held sentiment that there was not enough staff to handle the increased volume plus the greater demands of coordination across campuses:

> We didn't get a lot of extra treatment rooms, more staff, more work areas, a bigger waiting room. I mean, they just said suck it up. You're now going to take care of all of these patients. Their records are at the other hospital. Their doctor is at the other hospital. Their nurse is at the other hospital, down the street. And we're going to pretend that it's not down the street, and you're going to take care of all of them. And it's been a disaster.

"We don't do very good at it," Harris observed, as she described the shortcomings of the "patchwork" measures taken by the hospital to alleviate the workload in the ED.

"Even though on paper it looks like they have given us a few extra little helping hands, on a day-to-day basis it's not there," she explained. Although "they've given us something they call the practice assistants, who are supposed to help us," Harris continued, "it's not a fully staffed position. When they call in sick and [their positions are] not filled, and they go on breaks and no one covers them. . . . So, it doesn't really work."

"And they've made our housekeepers transport patients now. Well, okay, we have more transporters, maybe. But we don't have any housekeepers because they're pushing the stretchers. So instead of adding more transport people they said, 'Well, let the housekeepers do it.' But they didn't add more housekeepers." Harris concluded wearily, "So all those things, on paper, sort of looked like they addressed the problem, but it doesn't work" (June 1999).

In the ED, the unit coordinators and the personnel who stocked the rooms were being trained to be practice assistants, to take on some of the tasks that the nurses did. This, however, left fewer people to cover their other duties—manning the phones, stocking supplies, and keeping track of patient records. A housekeeper transporting a patient to a unit upstairs could not simultaneously prepare the now empty room for the next patient—sweeping, making the bed, disposing of trash. In the rush to accomplish everything at once, things would be missed. Garbage cans overflowed, and newly made beds lacked pillows (Fieldnotes, June 1999).

Nurses scrambled to fill the consequent gaps in service. A nurse manager from another unit explained that changes in one department often had consequences for nurses' work. "Everybody redesigns the work," she said. "Someone is always saying, 'Oh, we have this new guideline' or 'We have this new protocol we want to try' or 'We're not going to do this anymore.' So then you realize that 'Oh, that had a ripple effect on us.' That becomes problematic" (February 1999). To cite only one example, during the time of my fieldwork, the labs on the two campuses consolidated, as did pharmacy. As the new departments struggled to gain efficiency covering both campuses, there were slowdowns in getting test results and medications. Nurses, hurriedly trying to familiarize themselves with new protocols, paperwork, and schedules for ordering tests and medications, found dealing with these departments became more time-consuming.

In addition, the Genesis plan implemented budget cuts to a number of support services, among them dietary, transport, social work, and physical therapy. Nurses throughout BIDMC felt the full force of staffing reductions in these and other support services. A nurse manager complained, "If you're taking clinical support services away, you are impacting us as much as if you were taking nurses away. I mean, just adding on to nurses' work. I know they'd say they're leaving the nurse at the bedside, but they're giving them more to do" (July 1999). "It seems like now we're back to being the catch-all for every other service that hasn't kind of done their jobs," said a nurse in a focus group, voicing a common complaint. "Your time is being tied up with kind of nonnursing stuff that's important to the patient, but somebody else could be doing it just as effectively." She observed, "But nobody seems to be. And I don't know where the ball has been dropped. . . . These other services need to follow up. . . . Somewhere along the line the ball is kind of laying dead on the field, and nobody is picking it up. So we end up doing it" (Focus Group, August 1999).

In a second focus group, nurses agreed, "a huge portion of your job is making sure that everybody else does theirs" (August 1999). In yet another focus group, nurses raised the same issue: "There are some days I feel like I don't do my job because I'm doing everybody else's, and it's too bad. . . . And those are the days that you just do the minimum. You try to do the best you can with the time you have" (August 1999). All these nurses complained that when other services, which were also spread very thin, did not do their jobs, nurses had to pick up the slack.

"It is the nature of the humanistic caring work, and you have to do whatever needs to be done for the patient, even if it's not your job," a nurse administrator explained. "And it's always the nurse—because she's the one that's there, that has to make the systems work. When they don't work, she's the one that has to deal with the work-around. And part of the work is the work-arounds. And that takes time" (April 1999).

This nurse administrator tempered her remarks by insisting that nurses have always been a dissatisfied lot: "I've been a nurse for a long time now, twenty-five years, and we always talk about the systems not working, and not getting supplies, and the medication system is not working. And we can improve them, but systems don't always work, no matter how good they are" (April 1999). This dismissal of current complaints, however, flies in the face of the record of the former Beth Israel, which prided itself on giving nurses the support they needed and which, from many accounts, delivered on that promise.

At the time of my fieldwork, the multiple, simultaneous changes to staffing and to support services did indeed create new problems. As one nurse observed, "Once again, it comes back to an issue of poverty. If you don't have enough people to do the job, then you can't do the extra jobs" (July 1997). Nurses thought they simply did not have enough people to perform the daily work of caring for patients, let alone the extra work created by leaner support services and new systems.

In the ED, the nurses scrambled to cover gaps in service. In the frenetic activity of treating an incoming, acute patient, nurses often reached for supplies that were not placed where they were supposed to be. The nurse then left the room and ran down the hall to the supply closet, only to find there was no surgical gauze, syringe, or whatever item she needed there either. If she could not find the necessary item, which she had already interrupted her patient's care to search for, then she had to generate an order to restock it—a job that was supposed to have been performed by someone else. If this was not time-consuming enough, nurses often answered the ever-ringing phones and took messages or paged the requisite parties— another job that belonged to someone else—while preparing for the next patient or updating notes on patients (Fieldnotes, June and July, 1999).

Even without the increased patient volume, the ED staff would have had to deal with an increase in workload due to the extra steps involved in learning the new hospital systems or working with unfamiliar parties in other departments. Harris described the drain from all of the changes: "Everybody says everybody is resistant to change, and maybe that's true. But I think that there is a limit to how many changes you can have at once. Particularly if you change a system and then, in a few weeks, find that it didn't work so you change it again. And then you change it again."

"Over the last two and a half years, since we merged with the emergency room across the street," Harris emphasized, "our systems have changed over and over and over again—so often that nobody that works here knows how any of it works!" Harris explained that she had worked at Beth Israel for many years and prided herself on her system knowledge. Now, she said, "Every system that we use is different. How we give a report is different. How we document on the computer is different. How we get our medicines is different. . . . [E]very little thing we do has been changed in the last two years."

Adapting to the constant, numerous changes compromised her own and her fellow nurses' ability to perform their work. None of them, Harris said, could answer basic questions, fundamental to the ED's smooth operation, like "'Where is this kept? How do you get this? How do you fix this problem?' Everybody says, 'I don't know.' Even if it were perfect, you know, they can't change it endlessly and have us be good at what we do" (June 1999).

It is hardly surprising that nurses had less time with patients and that there was an epidemic of slowdowns and delays. Staffing levels were not increased to help manage the greater workload. Without extra nursing staff, there was no way to compensate for ongoing changes in the organization and still deliver care to patients.

Nurses' Powerlessness

Emergency room nursing is high-speed, high-intensity work. Nurses deal with unstable patients, patients whose diagnoses may not be clear, whose treatment plans are constantly evolving, who are in pain and anxious. One of the critical ways they manage high levels of uncertainty is to create and maintain a sense of order within chaos. This helps them make patients feel safe and secure, even if patients' conditions seem out of control. In the newly merged ED, nurses felt they could no longer maintain their sense of order. Indeed, nurses perceived themselves and their patients as the victims of organizational change.

Nurses confronted not only the demands of an increased workload but also a population of increasingly dissatisfied patients. Nelson, another Beth Israel veteran, described the increasingly common interaction of nurses with emergency patients:

> The most common thing you will hear nurses say, the greatest frustration, is that they are constantly apologizing to patients: "I'm sorry I can't do this. I'm sorry you can't do that. I'm sorry you have to wait for this. I'm sorry you have to wait for that. I'm sorry I have to put you in an ambulance and schlep you across the street. I'm sorry this doctor is not calling back. I'm sorry, I'm sorry, I'm sorry." And the great thing, I think, is that they're still saying it. (May 1999)

For the nurses, who valued their relationships with patients and identified with their experiences, these constant delays and ensuing apologies were intolerable. In numerous interviews, ED nurses fought back tears as they described working conditions. Some felt that patient care bordered on being "unsafe" or "dangerous," while others pointed to a decline in the quality of the care being delivered.

"There's less consistency," Carrie Taylor, a nurse who had spent five years working the ED, said. "The nurses are feeling more rushed in getting patients through here. Patients are being left in the hallways and feeling more vulnerable in the hallway. If you're not feeling well, the hallway is the last place you want to be in a chaotic department. I think patients are unhappy and the nurses are unhappy because they're not able to give the time and the care to a patient that they wanted to."

"I think the nurses feel like they need to be able to advocate for these people, [but they] can't because they're doing too many things," Taylor continued. "They're taking care of a lot of other patients at once. And those patients are suffering. We're battling seeing as many patients as we are in a day, in less space than we need to do it. We're trying to rush sicker patients through faster. The care is not as good as it used to be. And it's disappointing" (May 1999).

In a separate interview, Susan O'Neil, who worked in the ED for fifteen years, emphasized that this was a new situation in the ED: "People suffer. And it happens a lot that it feels really out of control, and it feels unsafe. . . . We used to have backup. . . . We used to just have resources we could pull, and we just don't anymore—there's just nobody available" (May 1999).

Nurses said they were doing the best that they could, but they felt powerless to change either the daily breakdowns and problems within the ED itself or the hospital policies that contributed to them. Changes in nursing administration at BIDMC only strengthened these feelings of powerlessness. In the spring of 1999, the ED nurses, who had worked as part of the Nursing Department, were transferred to a chain of command outside the Nursing Department. At the same time, their nurse manager of twenty years resigned. In the interim, the nurses felt unsure of their footing in the hospital and the department. "It's not just that they have lost a nurse manager. They have lost a nurse manager, and they lost a nursing director, and they lost their connection to the nursing service," Nelson explained. As a result, nurses did not feel that anyone powerful represented their interests and could intervene to fix problems that affected their clinical work.

The nurses attempted to compensate for their comparative lack of influence and authority by having the doctors, who had greater leverage, intercede on their behalf. They heeded the advice of one of the nurse leaders in the hospital:

> Physicians are really our friends in this environment because, when all is said and done, physicians care about patient care. So no matter how much political fighting goes on, you can always reach consensus around the patient. So that's really where we have tried to talk about the strategizing. We need to hook up with our physician colleagues around clinical care. . . . I think the physicians are definitely our colleagues, and that's where I have advised staff to build the strongest relationships: "Find your physician colleagues." (April 1999)

Nurses adopted the language of patients' welfare in order to motivate doctors' efforts. Mary-Jo Delvecchio Good ([1995] 1998) discusses the way medical students, who possess little status, invoke the language of patients' needs to challenge the decisions of those above them in the medical hierarchy. Similarly, nurses avoided stating challenges in terms of their own professional knowledge or needs. Because nurses lacked the status of physicians, they took an indirect approach and spoke instead in terms of the "good of patients." However, as Sam Porter observes, "the effectiveness of [nurses'] voices is still stringently limited by the powers that remain in the hands of the doctors" (1995:92).

Lisa DeMarco, a longtime Beth Israel nurse who had only recently joined the ED, recounted her conversation with a doctor about how patients could be moved through the ED more quickly if the full diagnosis for admission could be made after patients had been admitted to the inpatient floor: "[The doctor's] guard went up, and she got very angry. . . . I feel sometimes the doctors forget there are people sitting in those beds. . . . They're so busy focusing on the medical aspect that they forget there's a person there, that's been on stretcher for six hours, and that's uncomfortable" (June 1999).

DeMarco's claims of greater sensitivity to patients' needs provided the grounds for questioning the doctor's practices and later the doctor's lack of receptivity to her suggestions. She expressed her sense of frustration at her inability either to comfort patients or to affect change in the department through her conversation with the physician: "That's the part of nursing sometimes that really is very frustrating for me. That I can't help the patient deal with that. Because I'm powerless, I can't send the patient to the floor any sooner. Or I can't get that test done any faster." Framing the problem in terms of the patient's concerns, DeMarco questioned "how much . . . respect there is between the doctors and the nurses" (June 1999).

The issue of respect contributed to nurses' sense of powerlessness and lack of visibility in the hospital hierarchy. Many perceived their powerlessness to be a result of their subordinate position, and they viewed physicians' esteem as a force that tempered their inability to control other hospital systems and departments.

While nurses felt dependent on the good will of physicians to facilitate or improve patient care, the staff did little on a daily basis to improve relationships on the unit. Feelings of powerlessness, frustration, and anger took their toll on relationships among everyone in the department. "Everybody is so stressed and unhappy that it comes across in how we relate to each other," Harris explained, "Everybody is so cranky that we bicker and push each other's buttons and are not supportive and nasty. . . . It didn't used to be like that. Everybody worked together. . . . It feels so unsupportive" (June 1999).

Claims of nurses' greater sensitivity to patients' needs, especially when offered in this environment of generalized frustration and hostility, invited anger from physicians and were ineffective in achieving the desired support, resulting in an increasing sense of powerlessness among nurses. In contrast, emphasizing the common goal that doctors and nurses shared could increase nurses' access to power. Nurses were encouraged to use the discourse of patient care to build a coalition with the doctors. Seeking help from physicians within the ED, they tried to improve processes and expedite movement of patients through the department.

In the spring of 1999, as the Genesis team geared up for its redesign of the ED, Richard Wolfe took the helm as the new head of the ED. Wolfe was appointed Chief of Emergency Medicine, a new title in the organization that reflected the establishment of "emergency medicine as a separate, free-standing department" and recognized clinical discipline (and that coincided with nursing's loss of this same status). Recruited from Partners HealthCare, where he directed the residency program at Brigham and Women's and Massachusetts General Hospital, Wolfe made it known that one of the reasons for his decision to join the Beth Israel–Deaconess ED was that it had "the best nursing staff for emergency medicine in the city."[2]

Nurses welcomed his appointment as an opportunity to emphasize common goals. They were optimistic that this new chief could both smooth over some of the tensions between doctors and nurses and improve processes in the department. What they hoped for was lasting change, not just the daily victories that the doctors on the units could, through their influence, win.

Over the course of several months, Wolfe had the nurses write evaluations of the attendings and residents working in the ED. Nurses received this request as a "positive statement," a message to the doctors that nurses' opinions mattered—"I value what nurses have to say about you" (July 1999). Nelson, a senior member of the ED staff, recognized the Chief of Emergency Medicine's efforts to improve processes in the ED: "We now have a director who is invested in this department and who is invested in the management of this staff. . . . I think in general the issues and the struggles around patient care have lessened tremendously." Although "there are still some issues around outrageous behavior" of the staff toward one another, Wolfe's strategy of having the nurses evaluate the emergency medicine doctors gave the nurses more leverage in their interactions with the doctors.

Nelson was particularly encouraged by the new chief's vocal support for the ED nurses: "He has been up and down the second floor [where the administrative offices are] talking about how good the nurses are here. He's worked in fourteen different Emergency Departments, and he has never worked with a nursing service this good he says. And he says that to the CEO, and he says that to the President of the hospital. And that can't hurt" (July 1999). The nurses took comfort in the knowledge that the

[2] "Moving Forward: Richard Wolfe Joins BI-Deaconess as New Chief of Emergency Medicine," *Our News, A Publication for Beth Israel Deaconess Medical Center Staff and Employees* May 1999: 1–2.

Chief of Emergency Medicine thought so highly of their practice. They thought that he sent a powerful message to the doctors in the department that the nurses should be valued for their knowledge and skill and that nurses had legitimate claims to influence and authority within the department. Hoping that his leadership could improve conditions in the ED and shield the staff from further disruptions, they placed their confidence in his ability to bring about beneficial changes.

Relationships with physicians played a central role in nurses' experiences in the ED. Nurses viewed doctors as wielding the power to create or overcome numerous merger-related obstacles. By offering or withdrawing cooperation and support, physicians facilitated or hindered nurses' work with patients. When nurses took an adversarial tone with physicians, nurses tended to lose in power contests. However, emphasizing the common goals the two groups shared could allow for a redefinition of the relationships between them, and lead to mutual influence and empowerment of both doctors and nurses.

Doctor-nurse relations in the ED illustrated systemwide problems. In general, the common purpose that employees throughout the hospital shared in caring for patients became obfuscated by restructuring-related resentments. Constituents from the two premerger hospitals perceived the postmerger hospital as an arena for power contests. Consequently, employees on the front line experienced increasing stress and anger from their own powerlessness to get things done. Hospital employees, moreover, suffering from feelings of powerlessness, took their frustration out on longtime colleagues in the same department. Crankiness and nastiness eroded once good working relationships and diminished workers' sources of support. This situation reduced the power available to individuals throughout the system as vying for power obstructed coordination and cooperation and made it more difficult for people, particularly nurses, to perform their daily work.

Nurses found themselves dependent on gracious physicians—for example, a new sympathetic Chief of Emergency Medicine—who graciously lent their ears to the nurses' opinions and agreed to influence the behaviors of others on the nurses' behalf. But this was no way to run things.

At the old Beth Israel, nurses' influence did not depend on the courtesy of a physician. The formal power of nursing in the hospital and the accompanying organizational culture that valued nurses' professional practice had guaranteed that nurses' opinions mattered in patient-care decisions. The formal system ensured that, although doctors had the final word, nurses had some sway over patient care decisions, if not in every situation, then in most.

With restructuring, there was no formal mechanism or structure granting nurses any power. In the conflict-riddled medical center, the eroding relationships between doctors and nurses meant nurses were now frequently rendered powerless over patient-care decisions. When their influence hinged, moreover, on the benevolence of a physician, this was not good enough.

5

Doctor-Nurse Relationships

Melissa Fortunado, a nurse whose first and only jobs as a nursing assistant and then as a nurse had been at Beth Israel Hospital, experienced great trepidation and sadness on the dreary Monday she and three other nurses closed the Beth Israel Cardiothoracic Unit, 8 Feldberg. Each caring for only one patient, the nurses rode in ambulances across Brookline Avenue to the Deaconess Cardiothoracic Unit, Farr 6, to complete the merger of the units from the two sides. "It was sad," said Fortunado, "I cried when I left the floor." As they were leaving, her patient's wife took note of Fortunado's melancholy and in broken English said to her, "So you are leaving this home and you will go to another one." "She made me break down," said Fortunado, who said she felt like an idiot because she could not stop bawling in the elevator in front of the patient, his wife, and the two ambulance drivers.

When the nurses and their charges finally arrived on the new unit, Fortunado was too apprehensive to enjoy or be responsive to the warm greeting they received. She felt stressed, wondering, "where do I go?" and "what's going to happen now?" How was she going to take care of her patients on the new unit? In her anxiety, she did not take a moment to relax and get the patient settled. Instead, she immediately blurted out, "He needs a new IV, and how do I get that?"

Even though one of the nurses from the Deaconess side worked with her that day and showed her how to do everything, Fortunado "felt lost. . . . I just had that one patient, but not having a clue of anything. It was just really weird." The sensation of being lost and of not knowing how to function on the new unit was shared not just by the Beth Israel nurses who had moved to the Deaconess unit but by the Deaconess nurses as well. In the consolidation of cardiothoracic surgery, both sets of nurses were subjected to sweeping changes to their daily practice.

Everything from how to order tests to where nurses wrote their notes on patients were different on the two sides of the street. In preparation for the June 1999 consolidation of cardiothoracic surgery, the nursing staff from the three merging units had to decide which practices to adopt for the new unit. One nurse manager oversaw all three units, and she started working with staff several months ahead of the move to prepare. Nurses from both sides engaged in lengthy discussion about which practices were best. However, the adoption of particular practices was, in most cases, driven by outside concerns, not the consensus of the nursing staff.

Consolidating cardiothoracic care onto one inpatient unit involved the merging of three units. The two units from the Deaconess occupied the same floor, Farr 6A and Farr 6B, also called the Step-Down Unit. The A-side, the larger of the two units, received postoperative cardiac patients requiring standard care. The Step-Down Unit, one hallway out of four on the floor, housed patients who needed more monitoring than the basic inpatient unit provided, but not intensive care. Nurses on the A-side cared for four or five patients at a time on the day shift, while Step-Down Unit nurses generally had a smaller load of three patients per nurse. Because the A-side patients followed more predictable patterns, there was a high degree of routinization, guided by the surgeons' use of standard medications and discharge plans for their patients. In contrast, the Step-Down Unit nurses developed specialization in dealing with their more acute and complex patients, and they exercised a high degree of nursing judgment in caring for them. Generally, the patients from the Step-Down Unit would be discharged to the A-side inpatient unit once stabilized and ready for more routine care.

On the Beth Israel campus, the Cardiothoracic Unit, 8 Feldberg, cared for more acute patients than did Farr 6A, but the patient load was similar. The 8 Feldberg nurses enjoyed a lot of flexibility in planning care for their patients, and they administered a wider range of drugs and dosages than the nurses on Farr 6A. The nurses on 8 Feldberg cared for patients as acute as those in the Step-Down Unit, but these "heavy" patients were interspersed with the healthier patients who would normally be admitted to Farr 6A. In line with the hospital's emphasis on continuity of care, patients would be sent home with an appointment for a "wound check" two weeks after discharge. The patients returned to the inpatient floor for the appointment. At that time, their primary nurse checked their surgical scars for infection, answered questions, and instructed patients about medications and daily activities. In contrast, patients discharged from the Deaconess units had a visiting nurse check their wounds at home.

The hospital, in consolidating cardiac care, decided to merge the three units into one location on the Deaconess campus. The plan consisted of closing the Step-Down Unit, merging 8 Feldberg and Farr 6A, and expanding this new unit to include the entire floor. The decision to close the Step-Down Unit was made without consulting the Deaconess surgeons who had utilized the unit and worked with the nurses on the unit. In response to the decision, the nurses and surgeons circulated a petition describing the unit as essential to the hospital. However, the hospital moved forward with its plans to close the unit. The decision, which was made before the changes to the Nursing Department were implemented, seemed to be based on the hospital's commitment to primary nursing.

By getting rid of the Step-Down Unit, the hospital dispensed with the differentiated nursing practice from the Deaconess, where rank-and-file nurses managed a predictable patient population through standards and routine while more skilled, experienced nurses managed patient needs that involved greater uncertainty (see Chapter 3). The A-side nurses would have to raise their level of practice to accommodate a more difficult patient population. Now, like the 8 Feldberg nurses, all of the nurses would work with the wide range of patients admitted to the floor. The Deaconess A-side nurses needed to learn new techniques—including delivering medications through IV lines and using some new drugs—to care for these more demanding patients. This training, delivered through a series of in-service classes, constituted part of the preparation for the merging of the units.

While nurses had no input into the procedures that would be used to care for patients—this was the purview of the doctors—they scrutinized other aspects of their daily work. The nursing staff spent months comparing documentation—order forms, reports, nurses' notes. The hospital had not yet settled on standard documentation for patients' records, which were very different on the two campuses.

On the Deaconess side, nurses' notes were kept separate from those of other care providers—so that they would not "clutter" the medical record. Nurses' care plans and patient assessments were kept in separate notebooks at the bedside and entered into the patient's medical record only after discharge. These notes tended to be rather perfunctory. After filling in a worksheet assessment form, nurses then sometimes jotted down a line or two about the patient's condition or care plan on the back of the form. The nurses tended to communicate verbally any important information about the care plan or changes in the patient's condition.

In contrast, on the Beth Israel side, nurses wrote free-form "notes" in the same section of the medical record as the doctors and other care providers. In part because nurses were aware that these notes were not just for their own use but for other members of the care team as well, this format placed greater emphasis on recording a patient's progress and on developing the nurse's care plan. The Beth Israel nurses' notes were generally more thorough and descriptive than those from the Deaconess, but this note writing also took more time.

Because the newly merged unit could not dictate the form of the patient's record for the entire hospital, the new unit maintained the Deaconess practice of keeping the nursing notes separate from the rest of the record. For convenience, they also decided to keep the assessment worksheet that the Deaconess nurses used. The nurse manager did not, however, want nurses to slip into the habit of recording the information to fill in the worksheet and then neglecting care planning or skimping on documentation of the patients' condition. Seeking to reinforce primary nursing culture and practice, the nurse manager insisted that nurses use the more detailed documentation practices from Beth Israel—but, paradoxically, in the separate record—to help them document the nursing care plans more fully than was typically done at the Deaconess.

For the Deaconess nurses, this required a lot more writing and time, a burden many of them found irritating and frustrating. They felt, furthermore, that the note writing could not replace the verbal report. "There's a certain essence with nursing that you just know something. You know?" one of the Deaconess nurses explained, "If I went out there and said to another nurse, 'That patient has that look. They just have that look to them.' And she'd say, 'Oh geez, okay, well, let me know if you need anything.' You can't convey that on paper. It's like their vitals are fine but something is just not right about them. It still needs to be communicated between the staff" (July 1999). The Deaconess nurses felt that the notes could not capture the implicit knowledge that nurses had about patients and could not replace communication between the members of the nursing team.

Nor were the Beth Israel nurses pleased with the new charting arrangements. "We used to write SOAP notes in the patient's chart, and right now those notes get kept . . . outside their room in that blue book until they're discharged," one of the Beth Israel nurses commented, "And then it gets put in . . . their chart. So nobody reads them. Sometimes it's hard for us to find out information because if we are going through the charts to find out information on the patient, the nurse's notes aren't even in there."

Other members of the care team—doctors, social workers, case managers, physical therapists, occupational therapists, etc.—put their notes right into the chart for everyone to see. With the new arrangement, no one, not even the nurses themselves, bothered to read the separate nurses' notes. When the notes only recorded vital statistics and nurses verbally communicated pertinent information, perhaps the exclusion of the nurses' notes from the chart was not such a problem. But with the fuller documentation of primary nursing and less reliance on team communication, a lot of important information would be overlooked if no one read the notes. "I would rather them be in the patient's chart because . . . we spend a lot of time with the patient, and we're assessing them all day" (July 1999).

In standardizing practice, the nurse manager worked hard to solicit the input of both sets of nurses. The hope was that both sets of nurses would be able to retain the most valued aspects of their practice when the two units merged. However, it was not clear that these two very different cultures could be easily reconciled, especially when the overarching commitment was to the Beth Israel primary nursing culture. Many of the Deaconess nurses thought that because the nurse manager came from the former Beth Israel, she favored the Beth Israel staff and way of doing things. In an interview, Jill Dailey, a nurse who had worked in the Deaconess Step-Down Unit, voiced the complaints of many of the Deaconess nurses when she said, "This, to me, wasn't a merger. This was a takeover of their clinical way of doing things. It's been extremely frustrating. It seemed like, I guess, the Deaconess way just was always the wrong way" (July 1999). The Deaconess nurses did not seem to grasp that the fundamental characteristic of the primary nursing model—notes in the chart, which signaled nurses' value to and full participation in the care team—had been lost.

While the clinical decisions seemed to favor the Beth Israel way of doing things, other decisions, in the spirit of compromise, favored the Deaconess practice. In particular, the Deaconess nurses stood firm on the issue of getting off of the floor to go to lunch and of leaving on time. The Deaconess nurses justified this practice by referring to an ethic of teamwork and camaraderie, by defining patient care as a team effort, and by insisting that it was important to care for nurses as well as patients. For the Farr 6 nurses, the practice of going to lunch and getting off the floor, even just for a few minutes, was an institution. Half of the nurses covered patients while the other half went to lunch together at 12 or 12:30. The Deaconess nurses on the oncoming shift also often coaxed the outgoing shift, "Just leave it; I'll take care of it. Go home" (Fieldnotes, March 1999).

Fortunado, a Beth Israel nurse, described how these two practices were foreign to the Beth Israel nurses: "Over there we never got out on time because we were always sitting and doing our notes after work. We hardly ever went to lunch. If we did, we'd sit in the back room and have a quick sandwich, if that. You know, half the time you were going home and didn't even go to the bathroom. It was kind of crazy. Over here it is still a little hectic, but we go to lunch everyday" (July 1999).

I asked Fortunado why she thought the Deaconess nurses managed to get out on time and to have a relaxed lunch but the Beth Israel nurses did not. She responded that the Deaconess nurses "didn't have to stay and do notes after work." To them, she explained, "This is a twenty-four-hour operation. If you didn't get to finish something, the next shift can do it." In contrast, the Beth Israel nurses "didn't do that over there. If you didn't finish it, you would stay and finish it" (July 1999).

When the two sides merged, they tried to combine Beth Israel's primary nursing culture with the Deaconess practices of handing off work to other nurses for a half hour lunch break or at the change of shift to get out on time. But these handoffs seemed incompatible with the Beth Israel nursing culture. The twenty-four-hour accountability of primary nursing made it difficult for Beth Israel nurses to hand off patient responsibilities to the incoming shift. They had developed a work ethic that required them to take few if any breaks and to stay until all of their care tasks for the shift had been completed, even if it meant staying late. Such self-sacrifice was, to them, a sign of their much-valued professionalism.

The Deaconess nurses on the merged unit observed that it was often difficult to get the Beth Israel nurses to relinquish their care responsibilities and that some of the sense of camaraderie had been lost. Dailey observed, "We used to have fun here. We used to joke around, and we used to laugh a lot. We would laugh with the patients." She observed that now that the Beth Israel nurses had joined the unit, "People don't like to do that any more. There's no real joking around. Everything is very serious, everything is very Nancy Nurse-y, kind of. Try to keep all the ducks in a row, and try to look good in front of the docs . . . I think we just had a very different culture" (July 1999).

Despite their differences, the two sets of nurses worked together amicably. "I think we work together very nicely," Fortunado commented, "They were available for questions from us all the time. I've never seen anyone lose their patience. That's a lot—to have a lot of new nurses on the floor at one time, not just one, asking questions constantly . . . just like trying to figure out the system. They were always very patient and more than willing to help, which helps tremendously" (July 1999).

Similarly, an observer of the consolidation process noted, "Since the consolidation of the three units, I've . . . seen the nursing staff really pull together. . . . I wasn't here for the actual move, that first week, but when I came back, that second week, you still heard a lot of 'East-West,' 'we-they.' . . . And now it's . . . 'Well, what's best for the patient?' And I hear less 'we/they.' And sort of 'we,' as we're a unified front" (July 1999). The nurses on the Cardiothoracic Unit hoped to combine what they valued in their practices. Despite some hard feelings and trepidation about changes, they had been able to reach consensus around patient care and strove to work as a team.

Deteriorating Relationships between Doctors and Nurses

Despite the good working relationships among the nurses, neither side was happy with the results of the merger of the units. The central problem was the disruption of the smooth workings of the unit. "It's very frustrating because they are both used to being very proficient. And now, whatever it is, there are glitches that are hanging them up" (July 1999). Some of these glitches pertained to mastering new systems. At the time of the consolidation, the computer system used to prepare discharge papers and check lab results was being updated for Y2K. Nurses needed not only to get acquainted with each other and adjust to new paperwork, but also to learn the new program.

Other glitches related to broader merger-related issues. For example, the pharmacy and the laboratory had recently merged. The nurses had to learn a new set of phone numbers, names, and procedures for ordering tests or medications. As one nurse complained:

> It can be frustrating not knowing who to call, how to get in touch with somebody . . . We've been here since May, and I still carry this [note card] around with me that has . . . all different phone numbers that I might need . . . It's getting better, but . . . sometimes you feel like you are not able to spend as much time with the patient when you are trying to figure out things like this, and that's frustrating, but it'll get better—I think. (July 1999)

Like nurses on the other units I studied, the nurses on the Cardiothoracic Unit felt less efficient and resented the slowdowns that kept them from patients. The extra running around and time required to do formerly simple tasks frustrated them. But they acknowledged, through their grumbling, that the situation was temporary and would improve.

However, there was another set of obstacles around which the two sides showed less optimism. Nurses from both campuses displayed equal concern about what they perceived as a deterioration in their relationships with the cardiothoracic surgeons, a problem resulting from conflicts that developed between the Beth Israel and Deaconess surgeons after the merger.

In 1998, prominent cardiologists from the former New England Deaconess and Beth Israel Hospitals began to battle. In the interest of cutting costs and merging the two sides, the surgeons were being urged to standardize their practices—to use the same medications, tests, equipment, procedures and discharge protocols on their patients.

One of the surgeons, Andrew Simpson, said in an interview that it should have been a relatively simple matter to choose from among the practices of the two groups; one only had to look at outcomes and then at costs. Simpson, who was involved in the standardization process, explained that the two sides agreed to pick the methods that delivered "the same [or better] patient outcome . . . and lower costs. We're going to decide it that way. That's it. We're going to do it. OK. Fine." Sound easy? It was not.

Even when the outcomes were the same and the costs were clearly different, the surgeons could not agree on a standardized practice. The surgeons who would have to change their practice would have to abandon established patterns that they had come to consider "sacred." Forsaking their practice—whether it was performing a certain type of diagnostic test or using a particular brand of equipment—would, they felt, be admitting that their way had been "wrong all this time" and, worse, that the surgeons on the other side "were smarter" (September 1999).

Compounding the sense of competition between the two sides was an unfortunate incident in which Robert Johnson, a Beth Israel surgeon and the head of cardiothoracic surgery, "misfired a scathing e-mail" about one of the surgeons from the Deaconess. He questioned his colleague's skill, "saying he would hurt himself slicing a bagel," and then "accidentally sent the e-mail to the surgeon in question."[1]

Even though it seemed some balance could be achieved—an equal number of accepted and rejected practices from each side—both sides continually responded to the selection of the other side's particular practice over their own as "a personal insult." In surgery, a discipline known for its big egos and arrogance, it was hard to believe that there was no value judgment, no smugness, when one side was chosen over the other. Al-

[1] Liz Kowalczyk and Anne Barnard, "Infighting Hurt Merger of Beth Israel, Deaconess," *Boston Globe,* 25 November 2001, A1.

though Simpson and others went to great lengths to explain that no, the choice of one method over another was not a value judgment or a comment on an individual surgeon's skill or intelligence, but rather a reflection of the "common goal" of doing "the best we can for the least amount of money," no amount of assurance was enough (September 1999). The two sides could not be brought to some mutual decision.

None of the surgeons could tolerate being told that their practices were "wrong." All were invested in seeing adoption of their particular practice. They grew increasingly angry at the obstinance of the other side. In the medical building, where both sets of surgeons had their offices, they indirectly hurled insults at each other, loudly sharing rude remarks near open doorways, so that doctors from the other team would be sure to overhear (September 1999).

Animosity between the two sets of surgeons created barriers to establishing a sense of collegiality and teamwork among the doctors and nurses on the merged unit. In the past nurses had known the surgeons on their units and enjoyed collegial relations with them. "You knew [the surgeons'] kids, their wives, what they did on the weekend." Patricia Loma, a nurse from the Deaconess campus, said, "You had a very different relationship with them. So, when you had an issue with a patient, you could call them at home, in the middle of the night, three in the morning. You were appreciated; they would trust you." These close relationships facilitated the sharing of information about patients and the planning and execution of their care: "You really felt like the patient was getting the best care because you were both on the same wavelength, you both knew when the patient was going home, what the patient needed. . . . And the patient really appreciated that because they could see it."

On the new unit, nurses' relationships with doctors from the other campus were strained. Loma complained that on the newly consolidated unit, "You get all these mixed messages because nobody is communicating as much" (Focus Group, August 1999). On the new unit, the nurses had not yet developed the close rapport they had previously enjoyed with the surgeons from their old units, and this detracted from their ability to work together as a team.

Surgeons from both sides became stubborn about the way they wanted things done and intolerant of the practices from the other side. The disagreement proved very confusing for the nurses, who straddled two different sets of requirements while still orienting to the new unit.

Nurses' patient load often consisted of patients treated by both sets of surgeons. Nurses had questions about the new sets of protocols; they needed to know how to do things and what to expect in terms of patients' responses. Instead of being helpful, the surgeons responded with hostility to their queries. In a focus group, Jennifer Meyers, a Beth Israel nurse, commented, "They get so defensive when you ask them, 'Well, why do you want to do it that way?'"

Seeking to understand the rationale behind different treatment methods was not idle curiosity. Such understanding was critical to the nurses, who carried out the doctors' orders and monitored patients. Meyers explained that because she was accountable for the care she delivered to patients, "I want to know why I'm doing something differently. I was told this way, and that way makes sense to me. I want to know why I'm doing it this way."

Her desire to understand and learn met a negative reception, she said, with the doctors "giving me a derogatory remark, or mumbling and walking away, and getting pissed off and all defensive when you ask them a question. . . . We'd like to know why" (Focus Group, August 1999). Although the nurses wanted to feel comfortable with the new practices, the surgeons interpreted nurses' questions as yet another challenge to their authority or as a deficiency in the nurses' knowledge or competence. Their reactions reportedly ranged from unresponsive to openly hostile. Both sets of nurses did not trust the doctors because they were not on the "same wavelength," knowing what the patient needed and why. At the same time, the nurses felt that the doctors did not trust them because they did not value their input enough to seek it or appreciate their questions.

Just as the surgeons from both sides became stubborn about the way they wanted things done and intolerant of the practices from the other side, they displayed intolerance if nurses treated their patients using protocols from the other team. The doctors wanted the nurses to adhere strictly to the protocols that had been used on their campus before the consolidation. Not knowing the nurses from the other side, they were not willing to budge—to allow the nurses some autonomy in deciding what to do—and accept elements of a care plan typical of the other side.

In an interview, Carol Larson, a nurse from the Deaconess, described a common occurrence: "I think what everybody is doing is just doing it the way that they were used to doing it." There could be some lag between the time the doctor made the order and it got communicated to the nurses. In the meantime, the nurses sometimes reverted to the treatment course they were used to using on their old unit. "So then what ends up happening is that when you have like a West [Deaconess] Campus patient being taken care of by an East [Beth Israel] Campus nurse—and it's sort of like well, 'I don't like it done that way.'"

The doctors would became angry at the nurses for using a different, though appropriate, protocol. Larson observed, "I think that everybody was sort of not trusting each other. Again, attendings [doctors] not knowing the opposite campus nurses, not knowing their abilities. So I think they might have been a little more protective of their patients and a little less tolerant of, 'Well, how come it's not being done my way?'"(July 1999).

Not only were the surgeons unappreciative of nurses questions about treatment, but they were not physically present to communicate with nurses about patients. On the Beth Israel campus, the nurses and surgeons had gone on patient rounds together every morning. Meyers described the benefit of this arrangement: "You met with them every single day on rounds, and you knew at 7:30 what the whole plan was for the day" (Focus Group, August 1999). On the new unit, the Beth Israel attendings rounded less frequently with the nurses, and, the rest of the time, the nurses met with the residents and interns. Similarly, the Deaconess attending surgeons, who used to be a presence on the unit, showcased their displeasure with the consolidation by limiting their presence on the floor. They now arrived unpredictably and less frequently, and their residents and interns populated the unit.

Relying on residents and interns, who were still training and working under the guidance of the attendings, was not the same as working with the attendings. In the focus group, a nurse complained that even though there were at least two residents on the floor at a time, one from each service, they refused to answer questions about patients from the other service. When a nurse had a question about an attending's patient, she would approach the resident and ask, "Are you covering so and so." If the answer was "no," the nurse reported, then the resident did not want to be bothered and refused to talk with her about the patient. She would then have to search for the other resident on duty, who might be in the operating room in the middle of a surgery and unavailable. Consequently, it could take hours to get an answer to a question about a patient: "You go six hours without knowing whether or not somebody is okay. It's stupid stuff. Some of it is so dumb. But you have to talk to the doctor and nobody wants to take responsibility for it" (Focus Group, August 1999).

A nurse responded "in defense of our poor interns," "They're slammed. I mean, they are just overwhelmed with the number of patients that they have." "They are just pushed beyond," another nurse agreed. Not only were the interns and residents overwhelmed by the number of patients coming to the new, larger unit, but the new crop of interns and residents had only just taken their posts in July, a month after the consolidation. Their lack of confidence and skill made communication with the attendings all the more important and its lack all the more keenly felt by nurses, who required information about patients to plan their nursing care and discharge.

A Decline in Nursing Practice

These strained relationships with the surgeons challenged nurses' ability to provide high-quality patient care. In despair, a nurse sent me an anonymous handwritten note, in which she confessed, "Overall, I believe the merger has had a negative effect on nursing care. I have seen my own nursing care decline in quality due to the changes." While she recognized "that the change in environment and systems leads to delays in providing efficient care," she identified other "road blocks" to providing high-quality care: "Equipment and supplies are not readily available. The physical layout of the unit makes providing care more challenging. The nursing assistants require a large amount of supervision." Even more serious in her estimation was the lack of collegiality with the surgeons:

> Prior to the merger, I delivered expert professional nursing care to my patients in a timely manner. I was much more satisfied with my career and with my interactions/relationships with physicians, surgeons, and

> other health care professionals. Since the merger, I feel less respected and valued as a member of the health care team. I would no longer describe my practice as collaborative. It is infrequent that I have an opportunity to discuss a patient or patient care issue with an attending physician. It frequently does not feel as though my input to the interns and residents is valued. I have heard residents describe . . . nurses as "confrontational" because of their approach to collaborative practice. (Anonymous note, July 1999)

In this nurse's view, the surgeons did not value her perspective or insight into her patients, and some even rebuffed attempts at collaboration, misinterpreting it as confrontation. This lack of collaboration and consideration from the surgeons stripped her practice of a meaningful component of delivering "expert professional nursing care." Nor did she feel she played as central a role in her patients' care, and this feeling, she said, affected her own attitude toward her patients. Her own and her colleagues' loss of commitment to primary nursing created, she felt, "a lower expectation to provide quality care to patients on the new unit. Nurses 'know' their patients less. Primary nursing is not a priority, and there seems to be less of a commitment to primary nursing. . . . I feel as though nurses are doing their 8 hours (or 12 hours) and that's it" (Anonymous note, July 1999).

She pointed to problems "knowing" patients and to an accompanying decline in the sense of accountability for the whole of a patient's care. Nurses did not plan ahead for the next steps in their patients' care and recovery. Instead, they put in their time, attending to whatever care tasks needed to be accomplished in the immediate future, and then let the next shift take over. "Everyday I discover patients who are being [discharged] who have no discharge paperwork or teaching [about their medications and self-care] started."

This anonymous nurse's comments hinted at the problems that this lack of planning caused. It left nurses scrambling at the last minute to complete what—due to the new computer system and discharge forms—had become a three-hour process. With none of the paperwork or teaching done ahead of time, when nurses had more than one patient being discharged, they barely had time to attend to patients' needs (Fieldnotes, July 1999).

The nurse concluded, "[N]o one is looking ahead. I find myself to be guilty of this, because I am running to keep up with the demands of my job" (July 1999). To this nurse, the twenty-four-hour accountability of the primary nurse had not been replaced by the twenty-four-hour accountability of the nursing staff. In her view, no one kept an eye on the big picture and ensured that care plans were followed and completed.

In interviews, other nurses echoed these sentiments. Dailey, a Deaconess nurse who had worked in the Step-Down Unit, echoed the sentiments of many of the nurses I interviewed when she stated, "I think that Nursing 101 has gone way down the tubes, way down the tubes in the past couple of months. . . . I'm constantly finding mistakes, people constantly leaving stuff for other people to pick up. And it's been very disheartening lately."

While she did not blame a lack of respect from the surgeons for the "disheartening" situation, she pointed to a lack of communication among members of the medical team:

> The way they're doing reports now, I don't know anything about these people. . . . I don't have time in the mornings to sit there and read a chart for forty-five minutes. . . . I'm relying on the other staff members to pass along pertinent information, and it's not getting done. . . . I just found out in rounds that one guy has probably taken a hit to his kidneys. And I knew nothing about it, or why, what his history was for those problems. I used to know these patients inside and out, head to toe. And I don't any more. That bothers me.

In addition to problems with "knowing" the patients, Dailey, like the anonymous Beth Israel nurse, also noticed nurses leaving tasks for others to accomplish, "There's just been a lot of stuff that's really gone by the wayside. It's frustrating, very frustrating. . . . Some of these patients are kind of getting lost in the shuffle of things, with things not getting done, things kind of get put off" (July 1999).

Both of these nurses confronted the same troublesome issues. The merger compromised the things that they valued most about their practice. Of central issue to both nurses was the way aspects of patient care fell through the cracks. Without pertinent information on patients—about their problems or the surgeons' plan of action for them—primary nurses found it difficult to plan appropriate nursing care. The surgeons, in their turn, rebuffed nurses' attempts to solicit information and did not welcome nurses' insights or opinions about patients. Moreover, the surgeons disapproved of any divergence from their preferred treatment, particularly if it reflected a practice from the other side. With little shared information and so many constraints on practice, nurses were limited in their ability to make independent decisions and to plan care. Thwarted in their efforts to collaborate with the surgeons and feeling that they exercised little influence or authority over their patients' care, nurses' sense of having twenty-four-hour accountability for their patients dwindled. With their practice reduced to following the orders of warring surgeons, nurses resigned themselves to putting in their time and leaving the remainder of their unfinished work for the next shift. As a result, continuity of care could be compromised, with patients "getting lost in the shuffle" and not having their needs met.

Resistance from the Surgeons

In a study of physician resistance to a hospital merger, Rothman, Scwartzbaum, and McGrath (1971) suggest that organizational restructuring may threaten the mutual accommodations between professionals and the bureaucratic organizations employing them. As power is called into question, those concerned with losing power oppose and resist organizational change. Compared to other professional groups in hospitals, physicians are exceptionally well-positioned to mount effective resistance and opposition to change: They generate revenue, account for the hospital's referrals and prestige, and occupy several positions on the executive board (e.g., Chief of Medicine, Chief of Surgery, Chief of Emergency Medicine).

When a merger or other organizational upheaval challenges physicians' commitment to their positions or employing organizations by somehow threatening their status, physicians may circumvent the traditional bureaucratic authority of the hospital administration. They may buck the regular bureaucratic channels, with negative consequences for the orderly "transmission of information and 'orders' bearing on patient care" (Freidson 1970:121). Indeed, in the case of the Cardiothoracic Unit, the surgeons thwarted the hospital administration's directive to standardize practice. They invoked their medical authority to continue the modes of treatment they had used prior to consolidation. Although the Beth Israel and Deaconess surgeons did not have the power to stop the physical merger of the cardiothoracic units, they were able, during the time of my fieldwork, to block the merging of practices.

In the first focus group that I held on the consolidated Cardiothoracic Unit two months after the consolidation, the nurses spent the better part of our time detailing how the lack of standardization was the biggest obstacle to delivering what they considered good nursing care. Nurses were very unhappy with the communication breakdown, aggravated by the extra work of treating the same problems two different ways, and worried about the effect the lack of coordination had on patients. "To me, I'm sick and tired," one complained, "To me, it makes me not like the job any more. Because I'm not doing my best. I feel like my hands are tied behind my back sometimes. Because you can give and give and give and do your best, but I just feel like we're roadblocked."

Another nurse concurred, "We feel the same way. We just feel everything is helter-skelter. But I just think people need to put on their brakes and get together, you know."

A third nurse agreed, "It's like it's maybe too much, too soon, too different. We need standardization, that's what we need. Standardization, across the board. And maybe the doctors need to talk to the other doctors. . . . Because we're all in the same boat."

Later in the discussion, another nurse echoed these sentiments, "I just think we can standardize. We just need a little direction from somebody. God knows who. And then get things underway." The nurses blamed the surgeons for the current difficulties on the unit: "It's trickling down. It's from a surgeon's point of view that things are so different. And a lot of them aren't willing to budge" (Focus Group, August 1999).

To protest the merger, the surgeons insisted that, no matter how unfamiliar, nurses follow the particular protocols the surgeon used when treating that surgeon's patients. A nurse could not decide, for example, whether a patient should be scheduled to return to the unit for a wound check (the former Beth Israel practice) or should be sent home with a referral to see a visiting nurse (the former Deaconness practice). Although both courses were appropriate, the choice depended on which attending had performed the patient's surgery, and nurses had no latitude to decide this and other care plan issues.

However much the cardiothoracic surgeons might have felt out of control of the events at BIDMC, they nonetheless retained control over the nurses' work. Restructuring did not change the fundamental subordination of nurses to physicians. As doctors' subordinates (Abbott 1988; Chambliss 1996; Freidson 1970; Macdonald 1995; Porter 1995; Wicks 1998; Witz 1992), nurses at BIDMC suffered the effects of doctors' resistance and power contests. Fighting among the surgeons changed the nature of nurses' subordination—from one of collaboration with the surgeon making the final decision about a patient's care to one of total domination of patient-care decisions by the surgeons.

For an outside observer, this shift is easy to miss. Suzanne Gordon (1997) explains:

> When nurses work closely with doctors, they often suggest the medication to be used or an alteration in the doctor's prescribed plan. But even if their input is accepted, it's often not publicly acknowledged. Only the doctor's orders—not the fact that the nurse may have recommended them—are recorded on the patient's chart. A nurse's participation in this aspect of patient care—and thus the collaborative nature of the health care enterprise—remains invisible. The written record, which reflects the formal chains of authority and command in the medical system, maintains the fiction that the doctor is solely in charge. (173)

Despite the sometimes invisible nature of nurses' influence in patient care decisions, the collaboration between doctors and nurses was a core feature of primary nursing practice. Nurses saw it as their job to advocate for patients, particularly when they felt that the physician should adopt a new course of treatment. In cases when doctors were not receptive to a direct approach, nurses took more indirect routes. At Beth Israel, where the nurses' notes accompanied those of physicians in the medical record, nurses could skillfully craft these notes about patients' conditions and lead physicians to what they considered the "right" conclusion.

On the new Cardiothoracic Unit, both Beth Israel and Deaconess nurses who previously felt that the surgeons on their former units treated them as trusted and valued members of the health care team, now found the surgeons decidedly unreceptive. With the attendings spending less and less time on the units, nurses lost the opportunities to influence patient care, even when the surgeon was one with whom they used to work collaboratively. With nurses' notes exiled to the notebooks near the bedside, moreover, nurses now had few opportunities to communicate their insights and information relevant to decisions about patients' treatment plans.

In an environment in which surgeons dictated the delivery of nursing care, nurses were desperate for the surgeons to get together to work out their differences and agree on a standardized practice. One nurse spoke for all when she insisted, "We're nursing, and we should be able to say to them, 'This isn't right. This is not working.'" Unfortunately, the nurses did not feel empowered to make such forceful statements to the attendings. Their response was to helplessly acknowledge that while the attendings "know what's going on," the nurses did not have the ability to get them together: "You're not going to get all four attendings in a room for nursing to talk to them. It's not going to happen."

When a nurse questioned, "Why not?" another answered, "Because they don't have the time, and it's not a priority in their life. They don't care. They think about cutting [costs], and it's not a priority for them."

"They want things the way they want it to be, and they don't want it to change. So it's their ideals," another observed.

The nurses had little patience for the surgeons' ideological struggle. "It's very different for all of us [nurses]," one said, "Because then we can never gel [as a team]" (Focus Group, August 1999).

Despite the fact that the discord among the attendings was interfering with the cardiothoracic nurses' ability to perform the work of the unit, they passively accepted these conditions. They complained to the nurse manager, but they did not take steps to approach the surgeons themselves or, as a group, to insist that the surgeons come to some kind of truce. Their complaints and concerns were voiced among each other and in the back room, not in a public forum or directly to the offending parties.

During the focus group, one of the nurses complained, "It's a very negative environment working here." Another agreed, "I've never worked with such a dissatisfied group of people in my life. It's sad." The first responded, "We'll blame it on the doctors, but I think they need to hear that. Because that affects their patients."

Like nurses in the Emergency Department, nurses on the Cardiothoracic Unit recognized that serving the patients' interests provided a common goal that could give them influence over doctors' behavior. However, in this case, the nurses rationalized that that was not enough.

Again, during the focus group, the chorus of helplessness and hopelessness played its one-note tune:

RN: Oh, they've heard it.
RN: I don't think they really care.
RN: I don't either. I think it's more of an ego or control factor. And this hospital is very much of a doctor's hospital . . .
RN: They don't go home and think about it.

Although a nurse had earlier observed that the doctors were trying to preserve their way of doing things because of "their ideals," nurses also perceived that the doctors refused to compromise because of ego and a desire for control. Nurses perceived that the attendings were not concerned about the smooth workings of the unit, as long as their patients ultimately got the care the doctors wanted them to have.

The nurses on the Cardiothoracic Unit pointed to the lack of teamwork with the surgeons as impeding care. The 1999 Institute of Medicine report on medical errors (Kohn, Corrigan, and Donaldson 2000) supports their perception. The report claims that between forty-four thousand and ninety-eight thousand people die in U.S. hospitals annually as a result of medical errors and emphasizes that, "[although] almost all accidents result from human error it is now recognized that these errors are usually induced by faulty systems that 'set people up' to fail" (169). The report, which provides little detail about the internal organizational factors that contribute to faulty systems, nonetheless emphasizes the importance of teamwork in preventing medical errors (173).

The nurses did indeed feel that they were being set up to fail by the lack of teamwork on the unit. A nurse observed, "I would never say the patients get horrible care. I just think that it's much harder for us to do our job on a daily basis." Without an immediate threat to patients' well-being, however, nurses thought they lacked the necessary leverage to change the surgeons' behavior. While the nurses believed the attendings would surely come together if there were a crisis in care, nurses felt powerless to influence the attendings to negotiate a standard practice in the interest of preventing potential problems.

The surgeons were so intent on retaining and exercising control over their own practice that the teamwork and collaboration that had previously characterized that practice became the first casualty. So consumed with their egocentric conflict, the surgeons did not consider how their little war might affect the nurses or patient care. They had lost sight of the fact that they did not deliver care for patients by themselves and that their orders were not in themselves enough to provide good care.

With the Nursing Department in tatters, the nurse manager had no formal authority backing her request that the surgeons work out their differences. Even though the surgeons were battling at the expense of patient care, nurses, even those who had been trained to be assertive advocates for their patients, felt they could do nothing more than wait on the sidelines—even as patient care suffered.

6

Not Enough Staff

During our focus group, the nurses on the General Medical Unit angrily recounted a recent conflict with management over staffing on the unit. As the evening shift progressed—from 3 P.M. to 11 P.M.—it became clear that the nurse supervisor planned to pull one of the three nurses scheduled for the night shift to work on another unit that was understaffed. With authorization from the nursing directors, the plan was to limit the number of patients on the General Medical Unit to twenty and run the unit with two nurses. This would create a minimum staffing ratio of one nurse to ten patients. But what would happen to their ten patients, nurses worried. These patients were real people, not identical little dolls who could be tucked neatly into bed and found, safe and sound, in the same position the next morning. The patients on the unit were very different, highly unstable, and unpredictable. "We had three people so sick, like they could go any time. And then they had to pull one of us [and send her to another unit], and we were only left with two nurses on nights. . . . It's unsafe." (Focus Group, August 1999).

Welcome, the nurses told me, to the postmerger budgeting system for staff called flex staffing. This program had been in effect since 1997. The concept behind flex staffing was that units would be staffed with enough nurses to accommodate their average patient volume. Units added nurses if the volume went up and subtracted them if the volume went down. At the old Beth Israel, patient units were staffed to accommodate their maximum, not their average, patient volume. If there were any open beds on the unit, then nurses would have a lighter patient load. The new system eliminated such "waste."

The new flex staffing system was not the former Beth Israel's system but the former Deaconess' system—adjusted to the new Code Green financial environment. At the time of my fieldwork, the hospital's seventy-three-million-dollar financial crisis had produced a paniclike mentality. The nurses saw this staffing system that was supposed to provide units with enough staff to accommodate only their average patient volume, rather than their potential patient volume if filled, as depriving patients of adequate nursing care and nurses of the time they needed with patients.

Under this model, nurse managers were now held to strict determinations or budgets of how many nursing hours of care a patient could get. If a manager exceeded her allocation for hours of care, she would be called into an administrator's office and asked to defend her decision. What nurses felt to be a flawed and problematic staffing system even at the best of times, now—at what seemed the worst of times—became, they said, a nightmare. This was not what the flex staffing model originally promised.

Flex staffing was loosely based on the models of lean production being used in manufacturing industries, particularly in the Japanese automobile industry (Appelbaum and Batt 1994). Lean production was an answer to the mass production system, in which buffers of inventory were often needed to make up for problems in the production process; lean production, through rigorous use of statistical method, sought to smooth the production process and thereby reduce the need for this excess inventory (Appelbaum and Batt 1994). Flex staffing was meant to mimic this system; in this case, staffing units was the problematic process to be smoothed through statistical method and extra nurses were the buffers of inventory to be reduced. According to what was touted as a model that would easily and efficiently allow managers to provide adequate supplies of nurses to meet patient needs, units would be provided with an accounting of their average number of patients. This average would then be used to determine how many nurses were needed on a particular shift. The model required that nurses be added if the average volume went up—by calling nurses in from home or pulling them off other units—and that they be reduced if the volume went down—by canceling a nurse's shift or sending her to a unit that required more nurses. The average number of patients at night was used to determine the staffing budget for each unit.

Before the financial crunch, nurse managers from both campuses had identified a number of problems with the flex staffing system related to calculating the average number of patients on the unit. Patient volume on a unit fluctuated throughout the day, especially in the afternoons when there tended to be a large volume of discharges and admissions around the same time. The average census at night did not necessarily reflect either the turnover of patients on the unit or the maximum number of patients that occupied the unit on a given day.

The old Beth Israel staffing system involved staffing to accommodate the maximum possible volume on the unit. Then, there were enough nurses to handle any situation. In the new system, the units were only staffed to accommodate the average volume. While nurse managers found it relatively easy to "cancel" staff when the volume fell below average, finding staff to come in to handle greater volume at the last minute could be problematic. A nurse manager explained, "you can get into a really lousy situation. . . . It's tricky because . . . it's very hard to flex up."

This particular nurse manager struggled to keep within her staffing budget. She refused to staff based on the nighttime census because that would leave her too shorthanded. But she also did not staff to maximum capacity because that would put her way over budget. She staffed her unit "so that if you had [all your beds filled] you could work that day. It may not be your best staffing, but you staff so that it's safe that day and adequate." The problem was that "safe" and "adequate" staffing did not necessarily reflect the number of full-time equivalents allotted to her based on her average daily census, and the nurse manager frequently exceeded her staffing budget. She defended her decision to "overstaff": "I feel like I can't staff any other way because at any given point in the day, I'm going to be [full]" (February 1999).

Fluctuations in the volume of patients did not worry the nurses on the General Medical Unit on the night in question because management had agreed to cap the census at twenty patients. There would not be any new admissions during the shift if the unit had that many beds filled. However, nurses took issue with the proposed staffing ratio. They questioned management's expectation that one nurse could provide "safe" and "adequate" care to ten patients: "People are sicker . . . People that come in now, to get past insurance, they have to be deathly ill or doing very poorly to come in. I think the nursing job has gotten harder. I think it's more demanding. People from management have no clue."

Predicting Hours of Care

Management's calculation of what constituted "enough" nurses depended on the number of hours required for the *average nurse* to care for the *average* patient on the unit multiplied by the *average* number of patients on the unit. The problem with this system became apparent when the situation on the floors deviated from the *average* expectation. A nurse manager explained, "On average, we're budgeted for certain hours of care per patient. . . . Where it becomes interesting is that's just on an average. And there's no tool yet that says your patients on your unit, at any given time, are average. So it is the way you budget, but there's not really a very good way to measure what the inputs really need to be for a patient. So, it's tricky" (April 1999).

How many hours a particular type of patient needed was determined by first classifying patients with particular diseases or ailments into categories and then calculating the average number of hours that nurses spent caring for patients within the category (see Norrish and Rundall 2001 for related discussion). But what if patients in the same category deviate from this average? What happens when some patients require a lot more care and others a lot less? If a patient required more hours of care than the average, the nurse had to borrow hours budgeted for other patients to meet the above-average patient's needs. This balancing act would not present a problem if there were a sufficient mix of patients with higher and lower acuity in the nurses' caseload—in other words, if overbudgeted hours for some patients could compensate for the underbudgeted hours for others. Nurses at BIDMC, however, frequently had a patient mix skewed to patients who needed more care than the average.

Although the hours of nursing care had not changed in three years, the length of stay had decreased by almost half a day (0.4 days) on average. The half day that was cut out of the patient's stay represented the time when patients needed the least hands-on care and monitoring from the nurse—time that could have been used to compensate for the greater needs of other patients. As the length of stay grew shorter, nurses found they had less wiggle room to balance the needs of their patients; almost all of the patients needed the average hours of care or more. Few patients required less.

With the shorter length of stay, discharges and admissions were more frequent. The staffing ratios did not allow for the movement and bustle on the units. For example, at any one time, it might appear that a nurse had only five patients in her caseload. In fact, over the course of the shift, she might be responsible for ten patients—five discharged and five admitted. Trading one patient for another was neither instant nor effortless for the nurse, who had to bring herself up to speed on the different conditions and needs of each patient and complete the required paperwork for admission and discharge. The quicker turnover of patients added to the nurses' workload.

Another problem was the very concept "average hours" of care. In real life, the average hours of care are not usually evenly distributed from shift to shift over the length of the patient's stay. On any given shift, the patient might require more of a nurse's time and attention. Patients' most serious needs had to be dealt with as they occurred and could not always be either predicted or delayed. The assumption in the staffing ratios was that a nurse would distribute the hours of care required by patients in her caseload over the course of her shift. But if a patient crisis occupied her for the better part of her shift, that made it difficult to deliver more routine care to the rest of the patients depending on her.

In addition, the staffing ratios did not take into account the characteristics of the nurses providing care. One of the doctors I interviewed strongly criticized the concept behind the hospital's number-based staffing system:

> In a simplistic form [this system], says that we'll have the personnel we need to take care of patients when the patients are in here, but if the patients aren't here, we put them somewhere else, so we don't have to have them sitting around waiting. If you reduce that, what that says is that you have to have a nurse or a provider when there is a patient. The relationship with those two people is irrelevant; you just have to be there. That is the antithesis of health care. It has nothing to do with care. There's no relationship. (June 1999)

In other words, a nurse needed to be present to care for a certain number of live bodies. In this accounting system, nurses are viewed as interchangeable; it did not matter which nurse cared for a particular patient. A nurse's expertise in treating particular types of conditions, her rapport with the doctors overseeing the patient's care, and her level of skill and experience were all irrelevant.

The system of adding nurses if the number of patients increased and sending them home if it decreased did not consider the time required for nurses to get to "know" patients. The knowledge a nurse may have collected about the patient's unique needs and the rapport she may have built with the patient and the patient's family are not a factor in the decision to send or keep nurses. Thus, a patient's primary nurse could be floated—sent to another unit, whether or not she had worked there before—to "flex up" the staffing numbers on that other unit. Another nurse, who may not have had any prior connection to or information about the primary nurse's patient would need to take over that patient's care. The time that the primary nurse had already spent learning about the patient—time that had already been used in the budget of time for the patient's care—would now need to be spent again by the new nurse.

There is no allowance, moreover, in the budgeted hours of nursing care for differences in nurses' experience and skill. However, as Barbara Norrish and Thomas Rundall point out, "a simple task like inserting an intravenous (IV) catheter into a patient to administer fluids" will take less time for a nurse who is highly skilled and experienced in performing this task than for a nurse who has less skill (2001:62). Newer nurses are likely to be much less efficient in planning and implementing care than seasoned nurses, especially when the newcomers have little or no clinical support to help with these activities. However, the calculation of the ratio of nurses to patients did not consider these differences in experience and skill.

Finally, the staffing ratios ignored the myriad changes taking place at BIDMC. The hours of care did not increase to compensate for the additional workload nurses faced in dealing with restructuring. Nor did the average hours allotted for patient care reflect the additional time required to master new systems and procedures. Nor did they reflect the additional tasks that nurses performed to make up for the shortfalls in support services or to work around system problems and other obstacles.

The hours required for patient care at BIDMC, as in other hospitals, were "projected based on the care anticipated rather than on the care actually delivered" (Norrish and Rundall 2001:62) or needed. If a nurse had a full caseload of patients needing more than the average allotment of her time, only the most serious issues would be handled, and the nurse would not be able to address other concerns that were important to patients. Nurses found this situation frustrating. A nurse complained, "staffing has been tight. Some days it's downright ugly" (March 1999). Another asserted, "without adequate numbers, it doesn't matter how committed you are. You can't do a good job" (July 1999).

Meeting Patients' Survival Needs

Nurses on all six units that I studied frequently experienced pockets of time during the day when staffing fell short of need. At those times, their ability to deliver what they considered good care remained "just at the edges of your control" (Focus Group, August 1999). Nurses pointed to lack of staff, whether caused by having fewer nurses or the additional workload of filling in the gaps in other services, as having negative effects on them and on patients. A nurse described the toll on her colleagues: "They're just tired of the day-to-day dealing with bad staffing, working all day without having a chance to sit down, having unbelievable days, feeling exhausted physically and mentally when you leave. It's tough to keep doing every day" (June 1999).

In a focus group, another nurse also connected poor staffing with lower quality patient care and increased stress levels: "When there's poor staffing, it kind of limits the care that you get. You like to give good care, and you like to think you're giving good care, but at times you're not. You're too stressed; there's too many people" (Focus Group, August 1999).

On days when units were understaffed, I saw nurses rush around, sometimes frantically, trying to provide care to all of their patients. In a focus group, a nurse explained that on such hectic days, "you don't even know who else is on because you're running around going, 'Oh, my gosh! What do I do next? What do I do next?'" (August 1999).

With only a limited, and sometimes insufficient, amount of time to divide among all their patients, nurses were keenly aware that they had to meet the survival needs of all before they could give any "extra attention" to any one. "Everybody is just going at a hundred miles an hour, trying to just do the basic things that they can for patients," a nurse explained. She and other nurses identified the "basic things" by asking the question, "What does this patient need to survive this minute? What does this patient need to survive when they go home? And that's what we're concentrating on" because doing anything extra "means you're taking the survival time away from someone else" (July 1999).

Nurses perceived that they developed patient care plans in a haphazard manner, driven mostly by patients' immediate survival needs. "My patients get poor care all the time!" Susan Lazarus, a seasoned, Master's level nurse, exclaimed. "Any day I can tell you what I should have done and didn't. And the list is long. And it's because you end up triaging. You do what absolutely needs to be done, and the stuff that you should have done, or would have been good to do, doesn't get done." She fretted over the quality of care that she and her colleagues provided to patients: "I could give [management] every day a list of the patients who got poor care from me. I could also tell them that patients get better care from me than most nurses because I'm twenty years more experienced than most of the nurses. But that doesn't mean that things don't get screwed up on my patients. They're not as mobilized as they should be. Their symptoms aren't treated as well as they should be." Lack of time, she insisted, impeded her ability to use her finely honed nursing skills to plan and execute appropriate care for her patients. "I don't have a chance to discuss the plan. . . . So you end up with these kind of plans going along, just whatever is already in place. You keep up with that because it's something. And that's not good patient care" (July 1999).

As their workloads increased, nurses focused on the immediate tasks necessary to stabilize patients and were less able to focus on the "big picture" of caring for patients. What was left out? Nurses had little time for those activities that might promote recovery or comfort. A nurse manager described her staff as "really overwhelmed" and "task focused": "They do the [wound] dressings and then the Is and Os [reports on patients' intake and output], which I think they need to do. Then they hope that the patient won't want to talk or need any emotional care because they don't have time to do that. I think that it is hard for them" (April 1999).

Lisa DeMarco, a nurse in the Emergency Department, recounted a typical situation. "I had two very critical patients, and it was so busy that there was no other nurse to help me. They were busy with very sick patients as well. And one [of the patients] was a critical patient emotionally and the other was a critical patient physically." The chaotic work conditions in the Emergency Department forced DeMarco to choose between the immediate needs of these two patients. Setting aside something she felt very important, she focused on stabilizing the physically critical patient. "I think I gave great care to the person that was physically unstable. But at one point I was thinking to myself, 'Well, I'm being pulled in both directions. . . . I need help. I feel unsafe, basically.'" What was sacrificed? DeMarco was unable to offer any support to her other patient, who suffered both the emotional and physical pain of a miscarriage: "I could give nothing to the emotional side of the person who was actually losing her baby and didn't know what the process was all about. Couldn't do anything for her and felt very helpless about that" (June 1999). Failing to meet this patient's needs made her feel "helpless" and "unsafe." Nor was she alone. Many of the nurses on the units I studied shared similar experiences. In the survey I conducted, 73 percent of the nurses reported that they did not have time to attend to patients' emotional or psychological needs, and 65 percent stated that this lack of time happened on a weekly or more frequent basis.

A nurse complained, "I don't like the feeling of walking into a patient's room and saying, 'Here are your medications for the morning.' . . . And I'm thinking in my head, 'Don't talk. Don't talk. Just take the pills. I've got five people today.'"

Nurses wanted their patients to feel that their primary nurse was there to support them. At the same time, busy nurses hoped their patients would not call on them for conversation or emotional support because there was no time. "I don't want that to come across when I'm taking care of a patient, because patients can sense that," the same nurse said (February 1999). Hoping to keep up the facade that there was a relationship between them, even if she did not have time to attend to the patient's emotional comfort, the nurse did not want her patients to feel that they were unimportant to her or that she was too busy to meet their needs. "That makes you feel sad—just to think that that's what patients are getting," another nurse noted, worrying, like others, that her abruptness and frequent unavailability left patients feeling even more vulnerable and isolated, "I think it's a scary thing for patients. . . . As much as you very much try to hide how busy you are when you walk in that room—take a deep breath, slow yourself down, do what you need to do—but when your name is paged ten times during the course of the conversation, and they're saying a phone call is for you, they [patients] can't help but know that you're busy" (January 1999).

Neglecting Healthy Patients

The image of a precarious balancing act was one nurses often used. In a focus group, nurses described the way balancing the needs of the patients in their caseload led to neglecting the needs of healthier patients. "Sometimes I feel like I neglect patients." A nurse elaborated the thought process: "Oh, I don't have to go into his room, he's okay, you know." Another nurse agreed, "You're so busy with other people. You're kind of like, 'Oh, that one is alright'" (Focus Group, August 1999).

One evening Lynn Edison, a Beth Israel nurse who was working on the Deaconess campus, was on her shift and taking care of her by now usual load of five very ill patients. According to the assumptions built into flex staffing, these five patients would all get an average amount of care, eventually. In fact, "two of them were not getting any nursing care because the other three were taking all of my time. The two who were getting zero nursing care were asleep," she said, "but they didn't get evaluated, and it would be a good two hours between times that I actually laid eyes on them. That's not good nursing care, but that is the reality of the kind of situation" (February 1999).

Similar stories abounded of nurses having limited ability to monitor patients. "I would want to be seen more frequently, if I were a patient, than I am able to see my patients right now," said Eileen Hughes, another veteran nurse, "I find it a great relief if someone has a family member with them, sitting with them, who I know is at least watching them, is there with them, knows they are OK. It's just a matter of actually eyeballing them frequently and just looking at them, making sure they're safe in the bed." She added, worried about the consequences of such lapses in evaluation, "The doctor isn't there twenty-four hours a day and if you don't have the nursing care to pick up on x, y, and z, to call the doctor to come see the patient, then you can miss big problems." While she accepted the hospital's contention that it could not afford to hire more nurses, she exclaimed, "With the acuity, I just think we need more bodies . . . We need bodies to watch these patients!" (March 1999). "Neglecting" or putting off the care of healthier patients—those not confronting issues related to their immediate survival—compromised nurses' important role of detecting changes in patients' condition.

Nurses were concerned that flex staffing—based on a model used in industries that deal with predictable product lines and stable inanimate objects—was dubious in its application to the care of patients, who, they pointed out, are inherently unstable. Janice Reed, a nurse who had been practicing for a couple of years, described one supposedly "healthier" patient who was "fine" at the beginning of the shift. "She was basically just hanging out, waiting for a bed at Spaulding [a rehabilitation center]. And she was older, and she was [sitting] up in the chair."

But then, as the day went on, the patient hit the call light to summon Reed. "The first time she called she had to go to the bathroom; she couldn't get out of the cardiac chair [by herself]."

A little later, the patient's light went on again. Reed explained that even though she had seen the call light, she herself had not responded to the patient, "So, I saw her light on, but [then] it was shut off. So, I figured it was just something like get me a drink or whatever." Since the call light had been turned off, she assumed that a nursing assistant had been able to address what she was sure was a less pressing need.

It turned out, however, that the patient was trying frantically to get Reed's, or any other nurse's, attention. On this "busy" weekend, the patient tried four times to summon the nurses, "and four times somebody hung up on her." It was so hectic that the clerk at the front desk told the patient, "Somebody will be down. Somebody will be down," but in the bustle forgot to follow through by sending staff to the room.

Some time later, after Reed had dealt with what she thought were the more immediate problems of the other patients in her caseload, she finally got to check on the woman. What did she find? "She was vomiting for over like half an hour! She had a call for help, and everybody just kept hanging up on her!" And the nurse's aides had not responded, nor had they alerted the nurses.

Luckily, the patient had not been physically harmed by the lack of immediate attention. She had not, for instance, aspirated her vomit, which would have led to pneumonia and a stay in the intensive care unit. The patient had, however, been jarred by the experience. To test her nurse's responsiveness, the next day, Sunday, she was "on the light all day. . . . I felt like she didn't trust me. . . . I felt awful."

Like the patient, Reed had been shaken by the experience. As she recounted this experience during a focus group, her colleagues sympathized with a situation they felt could happen to any one of them. "Sometimes when things are so busy and you have so many patients, it's hard," a nurse said, "You feel like some things are out of your control, to a certain degree. You can't know what's going on with every patient at the same time. And you feel like you have to and you should."

Another added, "And when you don't something happens" (Focus Group, August 1999).

It was precisely this worry—that something would happen to a patient—that generated such frustration about management's decision to staff the General Medical Unit night shift with only two nurses.

Running the General Medical Unit with Two Nurses

These kinds of experiences, repeated day in and day out, made the nurses on the General Medical Unit feel that BIDMC management was out of touch with the needs of the patients being admitted to the floors. The nurses thought management's decision to run the unit with two nurses was, simply put, "unsafe."

The patient population on this unit consisted entirely of patients that nurses from a variety of units described as more challenging, demanding, and unpredictable than surgical patients. The precarious condition of several of the patients on the floor, nurses worried, could easily produce several emergencies during the night. But if only two nurses were caring for twenty unpredictable patients, whose so-called stable conditions could alter in a matter of minutes, how could these two nurses divide themselves between two—or even more—life-threatening situations? There would not be enough staff on the unit to handle such simultaneous spikes in need; nor would there be anyone to provide nursing care to the remaining patients on the unit, regardless of their level of need.

Not only were nurses worried about the potential for several emergencies among this group of patients, they also worried that two nurses alone on the floor would be unable to handle even one emergency. "You can't run a code with two nurses," one said.

"You can't even do chest compressions on a patient with two nurses," another echoed.

"Who's going to record? Who's going to get the cart? Who's going to push the meds? Who's going to stand at the cart and hand me whatever I need?" one of the nurses asked, almost desperate at the thought.

"We're talking seconds, but seconds count a lot to save a patient's life," a nurse summed up the sentiments of the entire group.

Nurses also worried about what would happen to the other patients on the floor if the only two nurses staffing the unit were involved in the emergency. Who would provide care to the other patients on the unit? Who would monitor their condition? And what if there was a second or even a third emergency at the same time?

Despite these growing concerns, the nursing administration insisted that other units worked smoothly, even during emergencies, with only two nurses on the night shift and that the General Medical Unit should not be an exception. But the General Medical Unit was an exception. Since the merger of the Beth Israel and Deaconess Hospitals in 1996, it had had a 50 percent turnover—a higher rate than any other unit. As a result, the majority of nurses had started working on the unit within the last two years and had limited or no previous nursing experience. The veteran nurses on the unit tended to work part-time or on the evening (three to eleven) shift. On the rotating day-night shift, the most experienced full-time nurse had five years of experience. Therefore, the most inexperienced nurses worked the day and night shifts, and, on any given shift, they might not have a more experienced staff member around for consultation. The inexperience of the nursing staff on the General Medical Unit posed a major challenge to the appropriateness of using the same nurse-patient ratios that other units, particularly those with more experienced nurses, used.

Back in February 1999, a nurse had told me that one of the big challenges on her unit was making sure new nurses felt comfortable around just the basics, like how to function in an emergency. She explained that a lot of resources were directed toward the basics of helping people learn to manage a cardiac arrest. Due to cuts in educational resources, she said, "We have to do it all on our own—developing, and learning, and making sure that we are meeting our educational needs."

By August 1999 when I conducted the focus group with nurses on this unit, staff development presented an even more daunting task. In May, six nurses quit within one week. Not only did this leave the unit with a shortage of nurses, but after the rollout of the Genesis Project, there were even fewer resources available to help the nurses train for emergencies. The newer nurses on the day-night rotation did not have the benefit of guidance either from clinical nurse specialists or from more experienced nurses. With few on-unit educational resources available, the nurses on the General Medical Unit struggled to feel efficient and competent functioning during emergencies, which, they said, were a regular occurrence on their unit.

If a bad outcome occurred, nurses, not the hospital administrators who set the staffing levels, would face the consequences. "They come to our floor and say, 'Oh, you can run two nurses on nights. Other floors do it.' And that scares me. It's my license. You lose your license, you're done." "That's your career." "It's the end of your job," another agreed soberly (Focus Group, August 1999).

Nurses felt a sense of responsibility to their patients. They also felt responsible for the unsafe work conditions that oncoming nurses could face if the unit was understaffed. As a result, they worked overtime, taking double shifts, to make up for any shortfall in the staffing ratios. "Nurses *choose* to stay. We have people that do doubles all the time. They stayed till the morning or stayed into the evening because they're short-staffed." "You feel bad dumping it," telling the oncoming nurses, "have a bad shift" (Focus Group, August 1999), a nurse explained.

Trying to exert some control over the situation, one of the nurses from the evening shift insisted on staying for the night shift so that the unit would have three nurses—a number the nurses agreed was the minimum required to handle an emergency. Edison, the nurse in question, was the hero of the hour. Why? Not only did she pull a double shift to help out her fellow nurses, but, in the absence of the nurse manager who had already gone home for the day and was not there to represent her staff's concerns, Lynn stood up to the supervisors, who tried to impose the flex staffing ratio that, nurses insisted, would have created unsafe conditions on the unit. "They gave her a really hard time for staying, but . . . Lynn wouldn't leave."

A nurse reported that the supervisor had become angered at Lynn's act of resistance, telling Lynn, "No, you don't need to stay" and ordering her, "Go home!" The supervisor reportedly told the nurses on the unit, "Well, everybody else can run it with two."

"Tell the supervisor to put on her nursing clothes and get on the floor if she wants to send one [nurse] home!" a nurse retorted, angered on hearing this piece of the story. The nurses in the focus group doubted that the supervisor, who was, in their opinion, so cavalier about staffing on the unit, would have been forthcoming with any support had the night nurses needed it; they doubted the supervisor would have rolled up her sleeves to assist them in delivering patient care.

A nurse complained, "It's frustrating. . . . You sit there and you talk till you're blue in the face. We can't do everything for these patients and not have enough staff to do it. But nobody listens. That night that we said we can't run the floor with two nurses, no one was listening."

A nurse added quietly, "If Lynn hadn't stayed, someone could have died."

The nurse manager had already gone home by the time the situation had developed. On arriving the next morning and learning of the situation, the nurse manager, who was accountable for both the staffing budget and the overall quality of care on the unit, supported her staff's judgment. She took seriously their conviction that two nurses could not run the unit at night, even with a census capped at twenty patients. She forwarded their complaints to the central nursing office and argued their position that this staffing situation was unacceptable.

The nurse administrators, however, did not increase the unit's staffing budget to allow for more nurses on the night shift. They held to their conviction that the General Medical Unit should be able to function with just two nurses as other units did.

I left the focus group aghast at the story the nurses related. Their sense of crisis was unmistakable. After the focus group, I ran into one of the nurse administrators. I told her, "The nurses upstairs are so upset. You should hear what they're saying." She responded, "I know what they're saying. Where do they think the staffing decision came from? It didn't come from nowhere. I know what they're saying." The nurse administrator had been part of the decision about the staffing levels on the unit. She, too, firmly insisted that the nurses on the General Medical Unit should be able to run their unit with two nurses on the night shift (Fieldnotes, August 1999).

"Good Nurses," Exploitation, and Turnover

Nurses have been socialized by nursing schools, hospitals, and professional organizations to feel personally responsible for the care and comfort of their patients. Kathleen Curtis, a longtime Beth Israel nurse, described the pervasive attitude about caring for patients: "Where I came from and what I learned, the Beth Israel philosophy, is what I always followed, is that the patient comes first. And it doesn't matter what time you leave. You treat them as if you have all the time in the world." "I don't keep that like I used to," she admitted, but "I do still believe that you get them comfortable, you answer their questions, you get them something to drink, something to eat if they want something." "You don't just say, 'Here's the bed, someone will be in,'" she said, "You say, 'What can I do for you?' if you know that they were in the emergency room for hours and it's not comfortable down there. So you try to make it comfortable for them when they arrive and give them a very good first impression." One of the things she often does is find the time "to say goodbye" to her patients before leaving for the day. "And I oftentimes regret doing it because you go to say goodbye, and they need the bedpan. Or you go to say goodbye, and they want a drink of water and a piece of toast." This act of caring often delayed Curtis's return home, but she saw it as an important part of her practice and the personal connection she made with her patients: "If you come in and say goodbye they feel like they're important to you. Versus just check off the stuff and go home" (March 1999).

Many of the nurses in this study shared the view that, as one nurse put it, practice resides "not in the institution but in the nurse. So it doesn't matter where you are," she said, "You can put me anywhere, and I can take care of patients." "In any unit, you always have a very wide variation in terms of who does what. There are people that just kind of go in and just want to punch a time clock: 'I will go in, I will do what it says I have to do, and then I will go home,'" she explained, "Then there are people who are doing extra or working and trying to do right, and you have that kind of variation because it is really personality variation and how people see their role" (February 1999). In a focus group, a nurse expressed a similar opinion, "Some people get in and do enough to get by. Then other people go the extra mile" (Focus Group, July 1999).

One of the most interesting things revealed in my discussions with nurses was how and where they located nursing practice. While their complaints defined nursing as an organized, professional intervention, dependent on institutional resources and support, they would frequently revert to a kind of default position, in which the ability of a nurse to really care for a patient was, in contrast, dependent on her own willingness to give of herself.

In another focus group, a nurse took this notion of practice as existing "in the nurse" even further. Not only did nurses decide whether or not to push themselves to deliver more comprehensive care, but they questioned themselves—and not the unit or the hospital or the larger health care system—if they did not manage to deliver the care they wanted to give: "People are hard on themselves. . . . We're doing the best we can; . . . it's still a pretty high level of nursing care that we're giving. We just sort of feel like you wish sometimes you could do more. . . . You feel so stressed by certain days. You feel like maybe you're not doing everything you can" (Focus Group, August 1999).

Even though the nurses sacrificed to give patients the care they needed, the nurses said they felt stressed and criticized themselves for not giving patients the best care possible. Nurses compared their effort to deliver care in a hostile environment to climbing Mount Everest, whose summit "you can't reach it. And it's frustrating and you get stressed." "If you don't get to that goal," nurses said, then they felt they had personally failed because they were not being "good nurses" (Focus Group, August 1999).

Socialized into the primary nursing culture, they had internalized their personal responsibility for delivering good care to their patients. When a nurse failed to hit the mark, she called herself a "bad nurse" but did not turn around and call BIDMC a "bad hospital."

Although the nurses in this study complained about poor staffing and other changes in the work environment, they failed to organize to try to change their work environment through unionizing or going on strike. Nurses individually shouldered the burden of struggling against their work conditions to deliver the level of care that they as professionals demanded of themselves. They exhibited acts of resistance to the limitations imposed by resource constraints by daily sacrificing their own comfort for that of their patients.

Nurses sped up their work during the day. Many of them worked eight or more hours at a stretch without taking a break. Nurses revealed that they would go almost whole shifts without eating or going to the bathroom. "It's not unusual for me to work a twelve-hour shift and not be able to eat lunch till four or five o'clock. We have days like that too, where you can't stop. And there are a number of days where you go without eating at all," one nurse told me (May 1999). "There are days you don't eat lunch until three or four o'clock, starting at 7:00 A.M. There are days you try to get to the bathroom by three, literally," said another (May 1999). Indeed, not having time to sit down for a moment of respite, to eat, or go to the bathroom was a topic of animated discussion in focus groups with nurses.

How did they manage eight- or twelve-hour shifts without a chance to eat or go to the bathroom? I asked nurses. One responded that twelve-hour shifts "are definitely tough because by five o'clock you've had it. You've really kind of had it. But what are you going to do? I mean, the stuff has got to get done. Sometimes it really seems like all those other priorities take precedence over your own well-being" (July 1999).

In addition to denying themselves breaks, nurses also stayed late to complete work rather than ignore the "little things" for which they lacked time during their hectic shifts. In an August 1999 focus group, nurses claimed that they routinely chose to stay a half hour or longer beyond the end of their shift to "see things through, to make sure it goes smoothly." Nurses might choose to stay late "if you have a late discharge or late transfer . . . , you have to stay and make sure everything goes through sometimes."

Another nurse explained that when the end of the shift came along, "people can still be on the bedpan, the dressings haven't been changed, which takes a few extra minutes to do." Nurses were clear that the decision of whether to stay rested with the individual nurse: "It's really personal preference" and "there's particular nurses that just won't do it."

Nurses also took extra shifts when it seemed that staffing on their unit would be insufficient. "We're really good about not letting it go short-staffed because that runs into being dangerous when you do that," a nurse explained. Finding coverage for sick nurses or flexing up when the patient census increased often involved asking nurses to put in extra hours after a long shift or to come in from home. "We don't get overtime; we don't get anything, so there is not really a benefit to someone doing it except for their being a good egg and not letting someone else down," a nurse elaborated, "and that's hard to ask people to do. Very difficult. Especially if you've had a really bad day and then you want someone to keep going" (May 1999).

Nonetheless, nurses cut into their own personal free time to spend additional time with patients. One nurse explained that she would strategically schedule her vacation and personal time to allow her to spend longer on her shifts and not get burnt out: "I'm exhausted, absolutely exhausted at the end of a shift, physically and emotionally, absolutely exhausted. And for me, I schedule planned time because I know I need the break, and that's what I have to do. . . . I really like my job, but I also know what my limitations are too. I think ahead enough to try to schedule planned time" (May 1999). Using her planned time to recover from the pace of her work day allowed this nurse to continue working at such a demanding job.

In addition, a number of nurses reduced their work hours from full-time to part-time or per diem work. Linking this trend to nurses' regular decisions to stay late, Curtis explained that she never worked a regular forty-hour week: "Forty hours is baloney; it's sixty hours, seventy hours. I used to come in at 6:30, 6:45 in the morning. And if I got home by five at night it was a good day. Sometimes it was six. It was crazy." "Part-time is easier for me because I enjoy coming in. . . . I work about three days a week," she explained, "Every day I come in I enjoy it, but I have a break. . . . If I get out at one in the morning [instead of at 11 P.M.], that's okay. It's one shift." Curtis claimed that working part-time helped her do "a little extra" for her patients: "[It] enables me to stay here. I don't think I could have done it full-time much longer" (March 1999). Working on a part-time or per diem basis enabled nurses to work more hours on fewer shifts without suffering the burnout that would result from doing a full-time schedule with so many additional hours.

New nurses seemed to burden themselves less with these kinds of expectations. Because they had not been socialized in the culture of primary nursing, they had lower expectations, which protected them from the strain of the tougher workload: "I wouldn't say it to many people, but I think that might be to their benefit to not have seen how we used to do it because they don't expect that from themselves. I often remember seeing them eating dinner, and I'm still running around trying to get everything done," observed Hughes. "How can I be doing this for ten-plus years and still not have my act together?" she wondered. "I think that you still try to do some of those things that you used to do that you really don't have to do anymore" (March 1999).

While more experienced nurses worried about deteriorating quality of care, newer nurses were more optimistic. In the survey I conducted across six units at BIDMC, those who had been nurses for less than five years showed significantly higher ratings for the quality of care delivered on their units than did veteran nurses. Management might point to such a result as evidence of veteran nurses' trouble adjusting to changing standards. However, veteran nurses could counter that these numbers reflected newer nurses' ignorance of the differences in the level of care. They could, furthermore, blame this ignorance on the decreasing support and resources available for developing professional practice. For veteran nurses, the problem was not that they could not adjust to a lower but still acceptable standard, it was that their newer colleagues had no referent for high-quality care.

In one of BIDMC's most successful, though perhaps not deliberate, cost-containment and cost-shifting strategies, nurses took it on themselves to maintain the high standards of patient care. The high expectations that they held for themselves, especially those nurses who had been trained to think of themselves as "professionals," compelled nurses to try to meet patients' needs despite resource constraints. Nurses' sense of professionalism and personal commitment made them ripe for exploitation. If resources were indeed too lean for nurses to provide safe care at a reasonable pace and within the boundaries of their shifts, then nurses' additional efforts and self-sacrifice allowed the hospital to realize cost savings at their expense. The hospital shifted the costs of quality out of the hospital budget and onto individual nurses, who paid in their own sweat, stress, and demoralization.

Insidiously, as long as nurses continued to push themselves to their limits to maintain high standards, the hospital administration could claim that the hospital budget made reasonable allocations for patient care. Administrators could ignore nurses' increased efforts and point to the continued quality of care as evidence of sufficient resources. Alternatively, they could recognize nurses' additional efforts but claim that nurses willingly took on the extra burden of delivering care that surpassed patient's actual needs.

Burning Out and Leaving

Despite the difference in assessments of quality, both new and veteran nurses were indistinguishable in their experience of burnout. Of the 147 nurses who returned surveys, 55 percent of nurses reported feeling emotionally drained by their work on a weekly or more frequent basis; 45 percent reported feeling fatigued on a weekly or more frequent basis when they get up in the morning and have to face another day on the job; and 28 percent reported feeling burned out from their work on a weekly or more frequent basis.[1] Although more satisfied with the quality of care, newer nurses suffered burnout, along with their veteran colleagues, in trying to meet the basic requirements of their workload.

Nurses expressed increasing frustration at their perceived inability to deliver the care that they thought patients needed and deserved. Nurses on all six units expressed growing discontent with their jobs. While 77 percent of nurses reported that they were satisfied with nursing in general, only 57 percent reported being satisfied with their current job. In interviews, nurses explicitly and directly connected this lack of satisfaction with changes in the organization. According to one nurse, "Like all of us, we

[1] These measures are from the emotional exhaustion portion of Maslach's Burnout Inventory (Maslach and Jackson 1981).

all loved our job. All of a sudden it's not our job any more. It's something else that you can't recognize" (June 1999).

The complaints related to the speed-up of nurses' work and their changing relationships with patients, but not to money. Nurses at BIDMC did not complain about their compensation. Their salaries ranged from forty thousand dollars for a new nurse up to eighty thousand for a seasoned nurse. In interviews, several nurses claimed that their high wages were one of the reasons that they did not plan to leave. "If I could find another job, that would pay me the same—because they pay me enough to keep me—I would leave. In an instant," a nurse declared, "And I'm an old time loyal BI nurse, but not any more. (June 1999).

Nurses expressed concern about finding secure jobs at other hospitals given the similar budget cuts occurring in other Boston-area hospitals. A nurse summarized these concerns: "I've looked at leaving. . . . I've looked at going to other hospitals . . . , but it's happening everywhere. And the concern is always going somewhere, being the new person in, after being here for so long, losing what I have. . . . And right now it's a tough time to make a decision to go somewhere else. You want that paycheck. . . . I have a job. That's how I look at it" (March 1999).

Despite the attractions of pay and greater job security from seniority, roughly one in four (23 percent) of the nurses surveyed claimed that they planned to leave their jobs in the next twelve months.

Whether they planned to leave nursing or just their position at the hospital, many of the nurses I interviewed strongly considered leaving their jobs. "It's not the most desirable place to work," Lindsey Marsh, a nurse from the Deaconess, observed, "I think it's going to burn people out. And I think the old-timers that have been here several years are going to start leaving; they already have. There's already three, four, five nurses [on my unit] that have gone on to explore different avenues. . . . I think they're going to have a faster turnover rate here now" (July 1999).

Another nurse described the situation on her unit, "Now people are leaving left and right from here. I mean, our staff is walking off the job. Last week somebody walked off the job, a new nurse. She had been off of orientation maybe two months. And at the end of her shift she said, 'I'm never coming back'" (June 1999).

Marsh walked me through her own decision to leave her job in the near future: "When you feel that you're not practicing safely any more or you're so frustrated on a daily basis, it's time to shift gears. Either go back to school, get out of nursing, or just leave. That's all you can do. . . . I, myself, am going to try to get into grad school this January. Only because I'm thinking long term" (July 1999).

Certainly hospital conditions were bad enough to drive talented, dedicated nurses away from the bedside—to other hospitals or to other types of jobs. The decision of many of the BIDMC nurses to reduce their hours or to leave nursing raised important issues, especially given the current nursing shortage. An administrator wondered, "What will happen? Will we have the best going into medicine? Will we have enough nurses to take care of the baby boomers?" (April 1999).

7

Was Quality Affected?

I'm scared to death to be sick. I'm scared to death for any of my family members to get sick because it really doesn't matter how good the doctors are if the nurses aren't there to pick up on things to notify the doctor about. (March 1999)

The nurses are unhappy because they're not able to give the time and the care to a patient that they wanted to. And I think probably things are being missed. I think patient care has suffered. (May 1999)

I used to believe that this hospital took excellent care of every patient, and I don't feel like that anymore. . . . The care is shoddy. It doesn't feel safe from a practitioner's standpoint. (June 1999)

At BIDMC and across the country, nurses' voices echo in a chorus of increasingly serious complaints about the quality of care in their institutions. Nurses are crying out at hospitals across the country as their workplaces transform in response to market pressures. The 1996 *American Journal of Nursing* patient care survey (Shindul-Rothschild, Berry, and Long-Middleton 1996) reported that of 7,355 nurses responding to their survey, only 43 percent thought that the quality of care they provided met their professional standards. Has hospital restructuring threatened the quality of care?

A recurrent theme in this book has been the conflict between nurses and administrators over whether the quality of patient care was seriously compromised by restructuring. It is extremely difficult to adjudicate between the two sides. Defining quality and what it means for quality to be compromised has become complicated in this increasingly cost-conscious medical marketplace.

Comfort and Quality

On one side, the administrators at BIDMC argued that quality standards were changing with the hospital industry's financial crunch. The personal bond that nurses at Beth Israel Hospital used to form with patients—spending extensive amounts of time talking with patients to get to know them as people and to offer emotional support and encouragement—could no longer be a primary factor in defining care quality. Administrators asserted that although nurses' modified, less personalized practice might skimp on patients' comfort and nurses' professional satisfaction, it still maintained patients' safety.

An administrator compared the changes taking place in the hospital with downsizing and consolidating to changes in the airline industry, a service industry subject to similar cost-cutting pressures during the previous decade. "The airlines . . . have gone through an enormous amount of . . . downsizing and consolidating. . . . Their safety record . . . has improved. . . . And their costs are reduced. But if you ask the average person who flies, 'Tell me about the experience,' it's unpleasant. When I fly, . . . I'm not happy, but I'm not sure I'd say I'm suffering."

The implication for health care was that while patients may find their experience "unpleasant," they were not "suffering." Apparently forgetting that patients who come to the hospital are already suffering, the administrator identified the caregivers, particularly doctors and nurses, as the ones suffering. While many aspects of care in hospitals "are very good," the administrator recognized "that the piece that isn't good is the hurry-up, the stressful environment of patients and providers. I think that nurses and physicians are having a very difficult time." In this person's opinion, the "difficult time" for nurses had to do with their relationships with patients: "When you are a nurse, really you don't want your patients to feel that it's an unpleasant experience, and you're the one that is not able to make that difference" (April 1999).

Administrators argued that in the new economic environment, the hospital simply could not afford for nurses to take the time to hold their patients' hands and to learn the names of their patients' children. They argued, moreover, that such niceties did not meaningfully affect the quality of care, which they defined in terms of patients' safety. Were there medication errors? Were people dying unexpectedly? Were patients experiencing more incidents of avoidable adverse events—falling more frequently because there was no one to assist or monitor them, getting more urinary tract infections because their catheters were not removed on time, or getting pneumonia because they did not get up and move enough after surgery? Although they firmly believed the answer was no—patient safety had not been affected—there was no direct, comparative evidence available from BIDMC.

In support of the administrators' position, the vast majority of patients at BIDMC reported satisfaction with the quality of care they received. BIDMC performed a survey of all patients who received care on inpatient units during April and May 1999.[1] Of the 1,197 respondents, 85 percent were satisfied with their hosital care: 56 percent deemed the care they received at BIDMC excellent, while another 29 percent rated the care very good. Additionally, 83 percent of respondents said they would definitely recommend BIDMC to their family and friends.

For a hospital struggling for its survival, an 85 percent satisfaction rating might seem more than acceptable. This statistic might represent a good balance of cost and comfort—especially when BIDMC managed to meet or exceed the expectations of so many patients while also reducing its budget. Hospital administrators might see this patient satisfaction data as a sign that nurses overexaggerated problems with patient care.

However, in nurses' daily experience, this same statistic could take on crisis proportions. An 85 percent satisfaction rating means that one in seven patients reported dissatisfaction with their care. In 1999, medical

[1] I do not have hospital data concerning the response rate, the differences between responders and non-responders, or the method of survey administration. Whatever the scientific merit of the survey, it was used by the Marketing Department in the summer of 1999 as an indicator of the hospital's successes and the need for improvement along particular dimensions. Moreover, the results were treated as representative of patients' experiences at BIDMC and were referenced in several interviews.

surgical nurses at BIDMC cared for anywhere between four (but usually five or more) and ten patients, depending on their unit and shift. Potentially, then, every nurse could have at least one patient with serious complaints about their care on every shift or every other shift.

Moreover, despite the high level of praise for their overall care, patients had complaints about their nursing care. A close examination of patients' survey responses on nursing-sensitive indicators point to widespread disappointment with aspects of nursing care that administrators might consider the comfort component of care. Almost a quarter of patients, 22 percent, said they were unable to discuss anxieties or fears about their condition or treatment with nurses. When asked whether it was easy to find someone on the hospital staff to talk to about their concerns, about one in four, 24 percent, said no. When they needed help getting to the bathroom, 17 percent reported that they did not always get it in time. The hospital staff did not do everything they could to control the patient's pain for 14 percent of the patients responding to the survey. According to 17 percent of respondents, doctors and nurses did not give their families or someone close to them all the information needed to help the patient recover. Finally, 13 percent of patients responding to the survey said that they were not treated with respect and dignity while in the hospital. On one or more of these questions, a full 50 percent of patients identified problems with their nursing care. These results suggest that half of the patients treated on inpatient units did not receive the type and amount of care and attention they desired from nurses.

For a nurse at the bedside, such daily exposure to dissatisfied patients could quickly create the perception that care was barely meeting patients' needs. Moreover, the central nursing office reported a 400 percent increase post-merger in the number of patient complaint letters received. This was in stark contrast to the situation in the late 1980s and early 1990s, when most of the letters praised the high quality of nursing and it was rare to receive letters with negative remarks (Interview, March 1999).

In response to the survey question, "What would you do to improve care at BIDMC?" many patients praised the nurses and the care they received as excellent or as making the difference in their recovery. However, 13 percent of the comments—almost all of them from patients dissatisfied with their care overall—pinpointed problems related to the nursing staff.

(Other complaints ranged from topics of their length of stay to the quality of hospital cuisine.) These complaints reflected the same shortcomings in care that troubled nurses.

Patients complained that the nursing staff was inattentive to their needs. Delays in receiving pain medication—delays that could prolong the unpleasant physical and emotional experience of pain and also postpone healing—provoked a number of complaints. A patient voiced a typical complaint, "When I needed pain meds I had to wait over 1 hour 2 times." Patients also pointed to mistakes in delivering medications. For example, "Floor nursing care was awful. I had two nurses during my stay that were attentive—the others missed medication times and did not respond when asked." Another patient reported being offered a roommate's medications on several occasions. In his case, each such occasion represented a near-miss for a potentially fatal medical error.

Patients also recounted long stretches of time in which they did not receive the attention they needed from nursing staff. Late responses to patients' call for help were a major source of dissatisfaction. A patient complained, "I could never reach a nurse; despite our ringing our nurse's light/bell no one came—I had to call the main number at BIDMC and ask them to connect me to the nurse's station." In another troubling example, a patient claimed, "I waited twenty-five minutes for a nurse to answer my ring when I was having an ongoing attack and needed nitroglycerin. I timed it. I am not making this up." For patients, not having nurses respond to calls for help in a timely manner could prolong pain or discomfort or could engender fear that no one would rescue them should something really be wrong.

Patients also perceived that nurses ignored "healthier" patients. A patient stated, "When I was very ill the staff took good care of me but when I was out of danger they ignored me. On several occasions I had to wait more than forty minutes for them to answer the nurse's light." Another patient reported that "the nurses were short staffed," and the patient felt treated "like a bother not a patient." Another patient was driven to hire someone "to sit with me to help as I could not take care of myself and the nurses were always too busy." This person observed, "The doctors and nurses are overworked and always rushing around. Both in the ER and on the floors." Such experiences could make patients feel that their nurses not only did not have time to attend to their problems but that they did not care.

While the Beth Israel Hospital had been world-renowned for its caring, several patients perceived their nurses at BIDMC as uncaring. A patient complained, "Some nurses are very impatient and unfriendly." Another pointed to the need "to educate a staff in actually 'caring' for a patient. Physically and mentally," claiming, "Other than my surgeon who was excellent in every way my three-day stay was a very unhappy experience." "Staff morale seemed to be low," another patient observed, "I felt people at many levels seemed indifferent to the care they were providing." Patients also said that they would have liked more contact with their nurses; in particular, they hungered for time to discuss the emotional aspects of their illness experiences with their nurses. A patient who described himself as a "a young healthy person who could advocate for himself" complained, "Other than the rare nurse; this stay was an isolating demoralizing experience."

For nurses, these complaints from dissatisfied patients were not trivial grumblings. Together, they provide a picture of patients, albeit a minority, who suffered feelings of being vulnerable, scared, and alone. Hurting, physically or mentally, they were dependent on a busy, harried nursing staff who did not provide them with either the medication or attention that they required and who could make mistakes in their treatment. While many of the patients' complaints pertain to the "pleasantness" of the their hospital experience, they also have direct bearing on patients' safety. These issues of physical and emotional comfort extend beyond smiles and hand-holding. Medication errors or delays, lapses in monitoring, and lack of information about one's condition could all make patients' experiences not only unpleasant but also unsafe.

Nurses insisted that any definition of care quality necessarily included providing *both* physical and emotional comfort to patients. The statement of purpose and philosophy from the former Beth Israel Hospital's Division of Nursing was still being used at BIDMC and provided a clear statement about the importance of "comfort": "We believe that physical and emotional comfort is a universal health need, the provision of which is an historical and fundamental nursing responsibility." The comforting aspects of care—those aspects that made care a more pleasant experience for patients—were regarded as a "fundamental" responsibility, not some frivolous extra. Although hospital administrators easily threw around the idea that standards of care quality had changed, nurses were not given any new directives about what constituted quality.

Nurses expressed great frustration at not being able to provide comfort care to patients. Shannon Malone, a Deaconess nurse, said,

> Where do you draw the line on making this patient feel better? . . . As long as I'm working, I'll never accept that someone tells me that I shouldn't be doing something for a patient. [What] if you were sick and you were in the hospital and all you wanted was for someone to give you a shave or to wash your hair and you were told, 'Well, I'm busy. I can't do that right now. That's not a priority'? That's just so unacceptable! . . . The patient only knows what's going on in their room and what's going on with them. They could care less what's going on two rooms down the hall, and you're their connection to the outside because the majority can't get up." (March 1999)

Nurses resisted the view that patients' comfort was an acceptable sacrifice to be made daily on the cost-cutting altar. Hospital patients, unlike airline patrons, could be extremely vulnerable and dependent. Some patients depended on the nursing staff—to eat, drink, wash, go to the bathroom, receive medication, change position—not just for hours but for days. Often confined by pain or illness to their beds, not all patients enjoyed the luxury of knowing that they merely had to weather another couple of hours before they could stretch their feet or get something to eat.

Questions about Safety

Nurses denied that comfort was the only thing being sacrificed. They challenged the notion that care was safe if less pleasant. Nurses saw the health care industry changes as more ominous than those in the airlines. "When you fly now the seats are smaller; they only give you peanuts; there's not as many stewardesses . . . ; sometimes they show you a video at the front instead of doing the demonstrations of how to do the safety protocols,"

Carrie Taylor commented, "And yet, people get safely from point A to point B. And it's a little bit cheaper. So, it's not as pleasant an experience, but it's not a horrible experience."

Consider, she suggested, the differences between an airplane and a hospital. If a plane flies safely, it is because the pilot and crew are still on the plane. In a hospital it is different. Unlike the pilot, the "attending physician is not at the bedside twenty-four hours with this patient." So who is there to make sure the hospitalized patient has a safe landing? While nurses are supposed to be the hospital's twenty-four-hour surveillance system, cutbacks in the hospital left them, like doctors, with little time at the bedside. Plus, Taylor stated, cutbacks in the hospital industry did not deny patients things that were inessential. "It's not that you're missing a full meal or that you're getting a video instead of the safety demonstration—if you're not getting the pulmonary hygiene [to] expand your lungs and get you breathing and get you up and walking and [to get] you reconditioned again, you're going home sicker. And you're going home less prepared than you would have" (May 1999). If administrators insisted on comparing hospitals to airplanes, nurses argued that they should get it right. Hospitals were not just cutting the airplane equivalent of hot meals; they were cutting the equivalent of routine maintenance on the plane.[2]

Had the appropriate data been collected, nurses fully expected it would have validated their daily experiences: Patients were suffering a greater number of avoidable adverse events, their recoveries were delayed, and many had repeat admissions to the hospital because issues were not properly resolved before discharge. Moreover, even if the data did not show significant changes in these measures, nurses at BIDMC would have argued that it was only a matter of time before they did. The nurses insisted that they pushed themselves to the limits to maintain an acceptable standard of care quality. Work speed-up and putting in overtime were the only way nurses thought they could continue to provide the care they thought patients needed. As a result, many of the nurses in the study exhibited signs of burnout and said they were planning to cut back their hours or leave their jobs. Nurses questioned how long they could sustain the high standard of quality their self-sacrifice afforded. Without greater organizational

[2] Susan Chamberlain Williams, September 2000.

support, nurses did not think they could continue to maintain the level of patient safety and satisfaction records that they had in the past.

These perceptions and concerns were also reflected in surveys conducted at the hospital by outside observers. A comparison of opinions of independent groups of nurses at the hospital, collected for separate research studies, before and after restructuring illustrate a significant decline in support for nursing practice. Surveys collected in 1986 by Marlene Kramer, in 1991 by Linda Aiken and researchers at the University of Pennsylvania, and in 1999 by myself provide information about changes in organizational arrangements over time at BIDMC. All three surveys include questions from the Nursing Work Index (NWI) developed by Marlene Kramer and Laurin Hafner (1989) in their study of magnet hospitals. The NWI queries individual nurses about characteristics in their current jobs. The responses are then aggregated to look at organizational arrangements on units or within hospitals (Aiken, Sochalski, and Lake 1997).

The data from 1986 correspond to what the nurses referred to as the "golden" years, before managed care and changes to Medicare reimbursement gained momentum (Guterman, Ashby, and Greene 1996). The data from 1991 correspond to the beginning of greater managed care penetration, when hospitals began to pay greater attention to streamlining operations (Guterman, Ashby, and Greene 1996; PROPAC 1997). In contrast, the 1999 results reflect arrangements during a time of dramatic changes in health care in general and at the merged hospital in particular in the late 1990s.

A sample of nurses at the institution in 1999 perceived their status in the hospital, their level of autonomy, their control over resources, and their collegiality with physicians to be significantly worse than did groups of nurses surveyed in 1986 and 1991, before the merger and the hospital's financial crunch[3] (Table 1).

[3] The 1999 results have been corrected using multiple imputation to correct for missing data (see Rubin 1987; and Schafer 1997 for detailed explanation). Listwise deletion would have limited the sample to 106 of the eligible 147 responses, leading to a loss of valuable information and potential inefficiency and bias in estimators (King et al. 2001). I estimated missing values using NORM (Schafer 1997; Schafer 1999). I imputed four data sets. The statistical analyses presented are averaged across the four data sets using Rubin's (1987) rule for combining scalar estimands (a function available in NORM).

Table 1 Measures of Organizational Arrangements at BIDMC over Time

	1986	(N=186)	1991	(N=72)	1999	(N=147)
Survey question	Mean	S.D.	Mean	S.D.	Mean	S.D.
Status						
"A clear philosophy of nursing that pervades the patient care environment"	3.46	0.58	3.69	0.52	2.60	0.74
"A chief nursing officer who is highly visible and accessible to staff"	3.13	0.84	2.75	0.82	2.03	0.95
"The chief nursing officer is equal in power and authority to other top level hospital executives"	3.48	0.59	3.81	0.51	2.56	0.90
Autonomy						
"Freedom to make important patient care and work decisions"	3.34	0.62	3.72	0.48	2.74	0.77
"Nursing controls its own practice"	3.40	0.61	3.74	0.54	2.47	0.77
"Not being placed in a position of having to do things that are against my nursing judgment"	3.33	0.65	3.31	0.83	2.91	0.77
"A nurse manager who backs up the nursing staff in decision making, even if the conflict is with a physician"	3.35	0.74	3.49	0.73	2.86	0.94
Control over Resources						
"Adequate support services allow me to spend time with my patients"	3.35	0.62	3.38	0.57	1.96	0.79
"Enough time and opportunity to discuss patient care problems with other nurses"	3.32	0.64	3.67	0.53	2.41	0.72
"Enough registered nurses on staff to provide quality patient care"	3.39	0.66	3.81	0.43	2.12	0.85
"Enough staff to get work done"	3.19	0.72	3.53	0.63	2.03	0.78

(*Table 1—cont.*)

	1986	(N=186)	1991	(N=72)	1999	(N=147)
Survey question	Mean	S.D.	Mean	S.D.	Mean	S.D.
Doctor-Nurse Relations						
"A lot of team work between nurses and doctors"	3.31	0.58	3.32	0.65	2.71	0.70
"Physicians and nurses have good working relationships"	3.27	0.53	3.27	0.65	2.88	0.69

S.D. = Standard deviation.

Note: Nurses were asked to rate—on a scale of 1 to 4—whether each element was present in their currecnt job. 1 = strongly disagree; 2 = disagree; 3 = agree; 4 = strongly agree. See note 3 for additional information.

In 1999, nurses reported significantly[4] less supportive arrangements at the hospital compared to the nurses surveyed in 1986 and 1991. All of the organizational arrangements that Aiken and her colleagues identify as important for nurses' satisfaction and safety, for avoiding burnout, and for patient care quality (Aiken, et al. 1997; Aiken and Sloane 1997a; Aiken and Sloane 1997b; Aiken, Smith, and Lake, 1994; Aiken, Sochalski, and Lake 1997), changed with restructuring to make the hospital a less supportive environment for nursing.

Comparing the ratings by these three groups of nurses conveys both a sense of the dimension of these changes over time and their magnitude. Control over resources shows the most dramatic decline during this period. Nurses in 1986 and 1991 reported having sufficient resources to spend time with patients, discuss patient care problems with other nurses, deliver quality patient care, and get the work done. In contrast, in 1999 nurses disagreed that they had sufficient staffing or support to meet any of these goals.

Over the past decade, researchers have also conducted a number of studies correlating organizational changes within hospitals to patient outcomes. Studies that explore the relationship between nurse staffing and

[4] $p < 0.05$.

patient outcomes lend credence to BIDMC nurses' claims about deteriorating care quality. While a 1995 Institute of Medicine report on the adequacy of nurse staffing in hospitals and nursing homes found an inadequate body of evidence to evaluate the relationship between nursing care and quality (Wunderlich, Sloan, and Davis 1996), more recent studies have rectified this situation. These studies demonstrate that higher staffing levels (Aiken et al. 1999; Kovner and Gergen 1998; Tarnow-Mordi et al. 2000) and a skill mix that favors care by registered nurses (Blegen, Goode, and Reed 1998; Needleman et al. 2002) both help prevent adverse events and promote better patient outcomes.

Additionally, after analyzing three million state and federal computer records, the *Chicago Tribune* concluded, "Since 1995, at least 1,720 hospital patients have been accidentally killed and 9,583 others injured from the actions or inaction of registered nurses across the country, who have seen their daily routine radically altered by cuts in staff and other belt-tightening in U.S. hospitals." The article asserts that "errors have intensified in recent years as working conditions have put more pressure on nurses."[5] Similarly, the Joint Commission on Accreditation of Healthcare Organizations (JCAHO), in its report *Health Care at the Crossroads: Strategies for Addressing the Nursing Crisis,* states, "Higher acuity patients plus fewer nurses to care for them is a prescription for danger" (6). JCAHO reported that staffing levels played a role in 24 percent of unanticipated events that resulted in serious harm to patients.

While organizational support for nursing at BIDMC had noticeably declined during the period when I conducted this research, nurses there still did agree, although not as strongly as before, that status, autonomy, and collegial relations with physicians were present in their current jobs.

Additionally, while BIDMC nurses did not feel that they had adequate staffing and support, the staffing numbers were significantly better than those in many other hospitals in the United States during the same time period. BIDMC's staffing system involved minimum staffing ratios of one nurse to ten patients on the night shift and fewer patients per nurse on the day shift, when patients needed even more care. In contrast, the Califor-

[5] Michael J. Berens, "Nursing Mistakes Kill, Injure Thousands: Cost-Cutting Exacts Tolls on Patients, Hospital Staffs," *Chicago Tribune,* 10 September 2000.

nia Hospital Association advocated adoption of the ratio of one nurse to ten patients as California's *minimum* staffing ratio for medical surgical patients—day or night (the California Nurses Association, in contrast, advocated a ratio of one nurse for every three patients as necessary to attract people to the nursing profession),[6] and many of the California hospitals protested that this ratio represented an undue economic burden for them because they regularly staffed with even more patients per nurse. This raises the question, while organizational arrangements at BIDMC had become less supportive of nursing care, how unsupportive were they really? And how much might this change in support affect care quality?

Changing Standards

For administrators, the fact that organizational arrangements at BIDMC had become less supportive of nursing only begged the question: While quality may have fallen in relative terms at BIDMC, how far had it fallen compared to other hospitals? A hospital administrator challenged BIDMC nurses' sense that care was not good at the hospital. The administrator argued that at a Harvard teaching hospital, a lapse in care would be a "pretty flagrant foul": "You're looking at above-the-average when you look here. So when people say, 'I'm afraid about my license' . . . No, that's not true. You don't understand. You've been here too long. You need to go out into the light." The administrator insisted that the nurses' standards were too high: "You need to talk to some of your colleagues who are nurses in East Overshoe and find out what kind of care they're delivering and what their staffing ratios are. See how often they get to see patients. See how long they have to wait for pain medication. See what the standards are out there. They changed. They're not the same" (September 1999). The administrator's position was that nurses at BIDMC were not aware of the changing standards in the hospital industry; they did not appreciate how good they had it. By this reasoning, even if there were some measurable declines in quality, they would be slight compared to other hospitals where the standards were not as high.

[6] Jeff Tieman, "No Agreement on Nurse Staffing," *Modern Healthcare,* 19 March 2001, 16.

In a separate interview, Susan Lazarus challenged the premise behind the administrator's comment. "You'd be fooling yourself to think that care isn't suffering." She challenged the notion that BIDMC needed to join the bandwagon of deteriorating care quality, "If an industry trend is bad, then does that mean that we don't say anything? Where are the health care executives standing up and saying, 'This is a bad trend. This is unfair. Patients are getting poor care in my institution'? I don't hear that happening" (July 1999). To Lazarus, it did not matter whether care at BIDMC was better or worse than at other hospitals. The issue, in her opinion, was that care had suffered at BIDMC and at other hospitals, and administrators lamely accepted and even perpetuated the situation.

A physician administrator confirmed the nurses' view that hospitals, including BIDMC, adopted troubling industry practices in order to survive: "Survival is key. I remember a couple years ago we had discussions about what would we be willing to give up of what we were in order to survive. How far do you take it? Is there a limit? Is there a point at which you say, 'That's it. We are not doing it?'" This administrator and clinician observed, "I think it is clear there is no point. We'll do whatever it takes to survive and be whatever we need to be. And for those who find it uncomfortable, they'll leave." According to this physician, such a situation had serious implications for quality of care: "I wouldn't want to get sick here or in any other hospital during the next few years. The key to health care in the United States these days is don't get sick" (June 1999).

Lazarus further highlighted the problem with hospitals' adaptation to the industry financial crunch when she observed, "It's not necessarily better to go to the hospital that has cut its costs enough to stay in business, instead of the one that was trying to do things right and went out of business. It's a little scary to think about the care you're getting in the ones that have cut their costs, including us" (July 1999).

In fact, she asked, how could the remaining hospitals claim that quality had not been affected by the industry changes? "When the priorities change, then nobody is even looking at quality. So it will be very difficult for me to see how anyone could say the quality is there. They wouldn't know if it's there because they're not looking for it. They're trying to stay alive." "At this point," she concluded, "I wouldn't trust family in the hospital without me. You can't assume that they're going to get any nursing.

And that's a nationwide trend. And it's not one that anyone in this industry should be proud of" (July 1999).

While nurses recognized the need for cost reductions for the hospital to stay solvent, they questioned the acceptance of current conditions by the hospital industry. They looked to hospital executives to fight changes that threatened patients, but did not see the efforts either in the industry or in their organization.

It seemed that as the hospital embarked on cost-cutting and reorganization of service delivery, it was basing its standard for quality of care not on some principled articulation of what patients needed but on what other hospitals in the industry were doing. When the majority of hospitals in this country are struggling with issues of cost-containment and competition, determining quality benchmarks based on their current practices promises a slippery slope of declining care quality. Questionable practices gain legitimacy not because they represent what is in patients' best interest but simply because everyone else is using them. In interviews, BIDMC administrators acknowledged that the standard of care had fallen, but they justified and defended the current standard of care at the institution because it represented accepted industry practice. Asked, "If everyone else jumped off a bridge, would you do it too?" BIDMC management in essence answered yes.

Conclusion

Across the country, health care professionals claim that sweeping changes in the health care industry compromise their ability to care for patients. They insist that an institutional emphasis on profit-maximizing behavior and productivity interferes with the relationships and activities that promote sound medical and nursing judgment and healing. Despite these indictments, restructuring and cost-containment efforts in the health care industry continue at a rapid pace. Professionals' claims tend to be viewed with cynicism and dismissed as ploys to protect professional power, jurisdiction, and privilege. The conventional management wisdom is that the danger to patients is exaggerated and that, in general, health professionals oppose and resist changes because they want to maintain their control over health care.

Restructuring, Relationships, and Resistance

What was the response of the hospital leadership at BIDMC to the concerns of the nurses in this study? Sitting in well-decorated offices, rarely visiting the units or shadowing clinicians or patients, administrators casually told me that there was nothing wrong with patient care at BIDMC—no higher rates of mortality, no significant drops in patient satisfaction. In fact, with 85 percent of patients satisfied with the care they received, they said, things actually looked quite good. The nurses simply needed to adjust their standards. The problem, they argued, was that nurses did not want to adopt a new way of working.

BIDMC's leadership was composed of intelligent, committed individuals, top-notch managers who had proven their abilities at top positions in other hospitals throughout the country. When I conducted my fieldwork, their attention and efforts were directed not on managing conditions at the bedside but on the daunting administrative tasks before them. Simply put, they had to save the hospital. Sifting through piles of data and reports and spending their days in a seemingly endless series of meetings with other managers, they worked hard to discern the best strategies to balance margin and mission. This was no easy task, and many of the administrators strained under the burden of making the gut-wrenching choices between service and survival.

In the middle of what seemed like life-and-death decisions for the organization, these administrators had little time to spare to investigate nurses' complaints about restructuring. It was no surprise to them that nurses might be unhappy about changes that gave them less time with patients. But the nurses would have to adjust.

In their quiet offices, seemingly a world away from the chaos on the inpatient floors and the constant din of patient call bells, it was easy to wax philosophical about the nurses' situation. Administrators did not jog up and down the halls with frantic nurses. Nor did they live with the daily consequences of their tough choices. They were insulated from the effects of their decisions to cut staff or to consolidate departments. It was a nurse, not an administrator, who had face-to-face contact with scared, vulnerable, or suffering patients whose care might be delayed, disrupted, or downgraded as nurses struggled with changes.

In an attempt to turn around BIDMC's financial situation, the hospital leadership brought in consultants to help them find ways to trim the excesses in the hospital's operations so that they could cut costs but still provide excellent patient care—goals familiar to many of the hospitals struggling under the pressures of increased competition and reduced reimbursements. These consultants, however, had even less contact with the reality of day-to-day clinical care and patients' needs than did the hospital's own administrators. They had little understanding, moreover, of either the history or role of nursing in general or its particular history at either Beth Israel or the Deaconess prior to the merger. One of the nurse executives told me that the "twenty-five-year-old MBAs" on the Deloitte consulting team considered Joyce Clifford (the former head of nursing at Beth Israel who became the top nursing executive at BIDMC) their "worst nightmare" rather than a valuable asset. The consultants, according to the nurse executive, "clearly thought that nursing was too powerful" and the hospital too "nurse-centered" (April 1999).

With the consultants' input, BIDMC management selected the same cost-cutting strategies that many other hospitals were using—leaner staffing, reduced support services, increased use of nursing assistants, shorter lengths of stay—and were in line with industry standards. To the managers adopting them, all of these changes in and of themselves seemed rather innocuous. Yes, they admitted, the net result was that nurses had less time to spend with their patients than they might have wanted. But when the hospital was losing a million dollars a week, everyone had to make sacrifices.

There was more to these changes than cutting costs, however. These changes initiated a fundamental shift in the hospital's view of the role of nurses in patient care. The hospital, in adopting the standard set of changes in vogue in hospital cost-cutting across the country, also adopted an implicit philosophy of patient care that was foreign to the primary nursing practice in place at BIDMC. The new emphasis on efficiency and productivity was incongruous with the personalized, individualized care that had become the trademark of professional nursing practice at the former Beth Israel Hospital.

The hospital leadership implicitly adopted the attitude that "a nurse is a nurse" when it implemented the practices of floating nurses—assigning nurses to whatever unit needed more staff whether or not the nurse had worked there before—and asking specialty nurses to care for unfamiliar types of patients without giving them the time, education, or support needed to help them safely care for patients. A nurse could care for any patient, the reasoning went. She could deliver the goods, whether or not she had developed any rapport with the patient, was familiar with the particular patient's situation, or had any expertise in treating the type of problems the patient presented. All she had to do was follow the doctor's orders for the patient's care, this attitude implied, reverting to a 1950s view of nurses as doctors' handmaidens. This attitude simultaneously minimized the importance of nurses' personal connection to patients and the importance of nurses' professional knowledge, expertise, and skill. As cost cutting also reduced the doctors' time for patient care, this attitude—one very different from the Beth Israel's emphasis on nurses' role as planners of care and advocates for patients—gave doctors little incentive to communicate with nurses, other than to give orders.

The expanded use of nursing assistants exacerbated the problem. While state regulation maintained that registered nurses are the only ones qualified to plan and evaluate nursing care, a nursing assistant could perform many of nurses' face-to-face, hands-on tasks so long as the registered nurses supervised the care and ensured nothing went awry. In this system of aides taking orders from nurses, who take orders from doctors, it does not seem like it matters who gives the direct care to patients—as long as patients somehow get their care.

With the use of nursing assistants, the nurses, whose role had been reduced to one of carrying out, but not questioning or influencing, doctors' orders, were expected somehow to plan nursing care intelligently and then delegate this work to the aides. But on what basis were nurses supposed to plan this nursing care? What information about the patient were they supposed to use—information they no longer had time to gather themselves, information doctors no longer conveyed to them, or information brought to them by an aide who had minimal training and education? Although emphasizing the nurses' role as a professional qualified to direct the work of others, this system simultaneously undermined nurses' professional knowledge and authority.

Administrators, while perhaps not cognizant of the devaluation of nurses' caring and professional roles implicit in these change, did recognize the threat these changes posed to the highly valued tradition of primary care nursing. They argued, however, that primary nursing practice was somewhat obsolete in the new health care environment. When most patients only stayed in the hospital for thirty-six hours, they said, there was no time for the close relationships nurses used to develop with patients. They harped on nurses' complaints about not having enough time with patients and basically pooh-poohed nurses' focus on their inability to "know" patients.

By "knowing the patient," nurses meant learning about the physical and emotional dimensions of a patient's illness, finding out how the patient responds to treatment and manages complex medication regimens, and discerning what resources the patient will need to cope with their illness and treatment regimens once they leave the hospital. Nurses admittedly did a poor job articulating the therapeutic content of "knowing the patient." But the pervasiveness of nurses' discussion and complaints about "knowing" patients quickly make it clear to any interested observer that they consider it an essential component of their work, not some social pleasantry that made their day more cheerful.

Instead, locked in their offices, surrounded by paperwork rather than patients, executives interpreted this concept of "knowing patients" as mere chit-chat and superficial friendliness. In the interviews I conducted, numerous administrators told me that the nurses could not return to the personalized, individualized care delivered in the Beth Israel's glory days, when there were ample resources to allow nurses the pleasure and satisfaction of cultivating personal relationships with patients.

One—a nurse administrator, even—trying to impart to me the inherent unreasonableness of nurses' ongoing lament, shared the example of an IV nurse who became impatient with her colleagues' complaints that they did not have enough time to know patients. Reportedly, the IV nurse boasted that in the span of the five or ten minutes that she spent with each patient, she still managed to "connect" with her patients. "Patients always remember her name even though they've only seen her once or twice. She's learned the art of how to develop that relationship" quickly (March 1999), the nurse administrator emphasized.

This example, however, is poignant for its irrelevance to the nurses' complaints. While it was, no doubt, pleasant for floor nurses if patients remembered their names or smiled, this superficial "relationship" had no bearing on whether the nurse was familiar enough with the patient's situation to provide the care the patient needed.

Overlooking the therapeutic value of nurses' relationships with patients, administrators insisted that the hospital could not afford to indulge nurses in the luxury of getting to know their patients. Nurses had to change the way they provided patient care.

What type of care were nurses supposed to give now? Not a single one of these administrators was able to present a compelling picture to me or, it appeared, to the nurses who worked for them. No one discussed what the new standard should look and feel like to the nurses providing this new kind of care or to the patient receiving it. The details of the new standard were left ambiguous. In fact, in the many interviews I conducted, administrators did not even attempt to present a picture of what high-quality care looked like in the new environment; they were still figuring that out and had work to do in that area, many said.

By default, it was conveniently left to each individual nurse to figure out how best to allocate the limited time and resources made available by the hospital to meet her patients' needs. Though perhaps unintentionally, this approach let the hospital administrators off the hook. If nurses claimed they did not have enough resources, administrators could argue that nurses found resources wanting only because they had not accepted the new, but never-defined standard.

Management believed that while it may have cut out some of the niceties or comfort-aspects of care, it had still produced a workable situation for nurses to provide good, safe care to patients. The hospital leadership had not witnessed firsthand the mounting sense of crisis, the dissatisfied and suffering patients, or the overwork and frustration of frontline nurses. Like administrators in many other hospitals across the country, the BIDMC leadership insisted that their hospital provided nurses with adequate resources and support to provide safe care to patients. But they never examined how restructuring affected nurses' ability to do their work.

By never asking the question of how restructuring affected nurses, they were free to assume that any problems the nurses faced were the nurses' own fault. Any complaints the nurses made about the quality of patient care at the hospital, moreover, could be seen as reflecting nurses' dislike of change rather than any danger to patients. These were dangerous assumptions that led to poor decisions.

BIDMC administrators dismissed nurses' resistance to restructuring as an expected and normal response to change. This understanding of employees' resistance—an understanding shared by managers in many other organizations in many other industries—reflected a flavor-of-the-month trend in the management field. Change strategists and leaders often present employees as resistors of change (Kanter, Stein, and Jick 1992), who, despite their protests, must be led and pushed through the change process.

Employees' resistance must be actively managed, such management wisdom tells us, by leaders with a vision of the organization's future, leaders who see the "big picture" that employees do not. This approach to employees' resistance led administrators at BIDMC—as it could have other administrators in other settings—to try to control resistance rather than to seek a partnership with its nurses.

Dismantling the Nursing Department is a case in point. Administrators cast the nurses, who were warning about threats to patient safety and care quality, not as partners in the organization's performance of its mission but as obstructions to restructuring. The hospital leadership sought to reduce and control nurses' resistance to changes meant to increase nurses' efficiency and productivity. With the dismantling of the Nursing Department, the administrators achieved their goal of reducing nurses' power to launch an effective resistance to restructuring. In a nonunion hospital, the move left nurses without influence over organizational policies or procedures.

The administration's move to strip nurses of their status and influence might be viewed as a victory given the hospital's troubles. Administrators were, indeed, pushing, if not leading, the troops through the change process and forcing them to accept changes. However, to the extent that the changes, as nurses consistently claimed, were diminishing care quality and threatening patient safety, everyone lost—the patients, the nurses, and the administrators. But the administrators never took the time to investigate nurses' allegations.

The administration's attempt, moreover, to exercise its own power over nurses reduced the power of the organization to provide care to patients. In dismantling the Nursing Department, the administrators alienated nurses, who came to believe that the hospital cared only about finances and not patients. In 1999, the relationships between nurses and the hospital administration became adversarial rather than collaborative. Had the administrators taken the time to address nurses' most pressing concerns about patient care, their power would not have been diminished. This would have been an important step toward fixing potentially serious problems that restructuring had inadvertently created in care delivery and toward gaining commitment to changes from nurses. At the same time, the nurses would have felt empowered; they would have felt that their voice mattered and that they had some control over the hospital's future direction.

What made matters worse for nurses was the ongoing conflict and hostility that still plagued BIDMC three years after the merger between Beth Israel and the New England Deaconess Hospitals and the problems involved in consolidating systems across the separate hospital campuses. In the hostile postmerger environment, infighting impeded cooperation and communication. These conflicts spilled over into the relationships between nurses and physicians. In the conflict-driven environment, many physicians dealt with inevitable power conflict by seeking to control nurses' practice. When uncommunicative doctors insisted that nurses follow their orders, nurses felt they lost their ability to advocate for patients and influence and contribute to their care. Deprived of their representation in the hospital and their formal seat of power, nurses believed they had no recourse.

In trying to control and manage nurses' resistance, the hospital leadership engaged in a self-defeating pattern of power play repeated throughout the organization—for example, in the behaviors of the rival staffs toward one another and in the relationships between doctors and nurses. In this dysfunctional pattern of behavior, one side tried to control the other. Decisions were an arena for power struggles, demonstrating who held power and who did not. Decisions—about emptying dumpsters, about admitting patients, about standardizing practice, about planning patient care, and about implementing restructuring—became battles, in which one side prevailed over the other, rendering the losers powerless. Had these decisions instead been cast as opportunities for collaboration and cooperation—as opportunities to meet a common goal—each party could have exercised some influence over the decision. Each party could have been empowered. And everyone could have benefited from the multiple perspectives and diverse sources of information.

What makes the story all the more tragic is that the changes that the administrators worked so hard to push through seemed to have made little difference in the hospital's financial outlook or chances for survival.

Fighting for Survival

In the early 1990s, when hospitals began to react to managed care, some were able to cut costs, and some enhanced their competitive position.

There was, however, little evidence of the overall effectiveness of their strategies and little thought given to their impact on the long-term health of U.S. hospitals. Indeed, since the early 1990s, strategies to manage cost containment and competition have not provided lasting solutions. Insurance premiums are still rising. American hospitals are still struggling to stay afloat in a turbulent market, and they are still searching for the next quick fix.

As of this writing in 2002, BIDMC is again under new management and looking desperately and hopefully at yet a new turnaround plan. Even with the merger and with the streamlining of operations undertaken with implementation of the Genesis plan, the hospital failed to move in the direction of financial recovery. In fact, in 2001, James Reinertsen was ousted by the board of CareGroup for not making changes fast enough either within the network or within its flagship hospital.[1]

The hospital board has pinned their hopes on the talents of a new CEO of BIDMC, Paul Levy, formerly executive director of the Massachusetts Water Resources Authority and a dean at the Harvard Medical School. His supporters hope that the man credited with cleaning up Boston Harbor will also be able to clean up BIDMC. The stakes are high. If he cannot deliver the necessary turnaround, BIDMC may be sold to a for-profit corporation. For a top-tiered academic medical center with such a distinguished history of patient-centered care and community service, this would truly be a tragedy.

What went wrong? The very restructuring strategies that BIDMC, following the trends in the hospital industry, adopted to solve its problems were themselves a problem.

BIDMC was not alone in its selection of a merger as a turnaround strategy, nor in its disappointment with the results. Mergers have yet to show their worth as a promising turnaround strategy for struggling hospitals. News stories about the problems and failures of several high-profile hospital mergers show the potential of this risky strategy to cost rather than save millions and to compromise patient care.[2]

[1] Liz Kowalczyk and Anne Barnard, "Infighting Hurt Merger of Beth Israel, Deaconess," *Boston Globe,* 25 November 2001, A1.

[2] Jennifer Steinhauer, "Hospital Mergers Stumbling as Marriages of Convenience," *New York Times,* 14 March 2001, A1. Duncan Moore Jr., "System Divorces on Rise; Unscrambling

Mergers often created more problems than they solved. In some markets, greater consolidation in the hospital population quickly led to intensifying competition among a smaller number of larger rivals (Burns et al. 1997; Greene 1992). This competition increased hospital spending as hospitals added new services and facilities in a "medical arms race" to become a region's top provider (Greene 1992:37).

Integration of medical staff and facilities, moreover, has been a sticking point keeping many hospitals from fully benefiting from mergers. In March 2001, the front page of the *New York Times* announced that most hospital mergers resulted in the joining of "legal documents and back-room functions only," not a merging of clinical programs.[3] Hospitals often underestimated the difficulties and costs involved in integrating staff with different corporate cultures and procedures.[4] In some cases, hospitals that had hoped to combine departments faced such difficulties due to clashes of egos and culture that they duplicated functions instead of consolidating them (Greene 1992). Conflicts around the integration of clinical programs seem to have provided the irreconcilable differences leading to divorce in three high-profile mergers: Penn State Geisinger in Pennsylvania, Optima Health in New Hampshire, and UCSF-Stanford in California.[5] Incompatible corporate cultures and competition among medial staff were cited as primary reasons for these merger failures and implicated

---

Deals Is Messy and Contentious." *Modern Healthcare,* 29 May 2000, 24. Steven Syre and Charles Stein, "Mergers of Health Care Firms Often Just Don't Work Out," *Boston Globe,* 12 January 2000. Barbara Kirchheimer, "Going Their Ways: UCSF-Stanford Ends Tumultuous, Money-Losing Merger," *Modern Healthcare,* 1 November 1999, 2. Scott Hensley, "Penn State Geisinger Pulls the Plug; System Leaders Cite Clashing Cultures, Inability to Consolidate Services and Cut Costs," *Modern Healthcare,* 22 November 1999, 2. Michael Lasalandra, "Deaths May Be Symptom of Medical Merger-Mania," *Boston Herald,* 7 June 1998.

[3] Jennifer Steinhauer, "Hospital Mergers Stumbling as Marriages of Convenience," *New York Times,* 14 March 2001, A1.

[4] Steven Syre and Charles Stein, "Mergers of Health Care Firms Often Just Don't Work Out," *Boston Globe,* 12 January 2000.

[5] Duncan Moore Jr., "System Divorces on Rise; Unscrambling Deals Is Messy and Contentious." *Modern Healthcare,* 29 May 2000, 24. Barbara Kirchheimer, "Going Their Ways: UCSF-Stanford Ends Tumultuous, Money-Losing Merger," *Modern Healthcare,* 1 November 1999, 2. Scott Hensley, "Penn State Geisinger Pulls the Plug; System Leaders Cite Clashing Cultures, Inability to Consolidate Services and Cut Costs," *Modern Healthcare,* 22 November 1999, 2.

in the disappointing returns of other mergers, including the Beth Israel–Deaconess merger.[6]

In most cases, the cost savings expected from hospital mergers failed to materialize. A study of changes in hospitals' finances after a merger showed only modest cost and price savings (Spang, Bazzoli, and Arnould, 2001), but not the dramatic turnarounds that inspired hospitals' merger-mania in the 1990s. Another study of ninety-two hospital mergers also concluded that, even three years after a merger, mergers failed to provide the hoped-for turnaround to struggling hospitals (Alexander and Lee 1996). Rather, merging hospitals enjoyed only incremental change, a slowing of negative trends in operational characteristics rather than a "radical reversal" (Alexander and Lee 1996). What is unclear is whether these slowing of trends represent an even larger boon to a hospital that might not have survived had it not merged; perhaps merging hospitals have faired better together than they would have apart. Additionally, these modest improvements might represent short-term gains, with greater benefits still to be realized once facilities integrate more thoroughly and the initial disruptions and animosities have died down (Alexander and Lee 1996; Lee and Alexander 1999).

In the BIDMC case, it is impossible to know whether the New England Deaconess Hospital or Beth Israel Hospital would have survived on their own had they not merged. It is also impossible to know whether, in time, the hospital leadership could have overcome the rivalry and animosities between the two staffs and successfully consolidated. Just when the hospital began to make progress in this area, the effects of the 1997 Balanced Budget Act hit. Already suffering from costs and losses related to the merger, the new changes in Medicare funding threw BIDMC deep into financial crisis. Although the hospital needed to invest resources and time in healing merger wounds, it had the benefit of neither. The hospital needed to act quickly and make draconian budget cuts to reduce its deficit and remain solvent. They paid consultants millions of dollars to help de-

[6] Jennifer Steinhauer, "Hospital Mergers Stumbling as Marriages of Convenience," *New York Times,* 14 March 2001, A1. Duncan Moore Jr., "System Divorces on Rise; Unscrambling Deals Is Messy and Contentious," *Modern Healthcare,* 29 May 2000, 24. Liz Kowalczyk and Anne Barnard, "Infighting Hurt Merger of Beth Israel Deaconess," *Boston Globe,* 25 November 2001, A1.

vise a turnaround plan to cut costs and increase revenues. But the resulting Genesis plan, a plan to reorganize and streamline internal operations, also fell short of its promise, as did similar plans in other hospitals throughout the United States.

While hospitals often reduced their labor costs in the short term through changes in staffing levels, skill mix, and reductions in support services, no evidence shows that these streamlining strategies led to savings in the long term (Aiken and Fagin 1997; White 1997). In fact, there is some evidence that trying to wring greater productivity out of employees increased hospital costs due to staff dissatisfaction, turnover, and adverse patient events (Robertson, Dowd, and Hassan 1997). Burnt out and dissatisfied employees quit their jobs, saddling their hospitals with the additional costs of recruiting and training new employees. More important, evidence suggests that these staffing changes impaired providers' ability to care for patients and resulted in a greater number of adverse outcomes for patients—medication errors, avoidable infections, and, in some cases, lengthier illnesses and even death (Blegen, Goode, and Reed 1998; Kovner and Gergen 1998). With reports of deadly medical errors linked to staffing inadequacy, these trends raise serious questions about whether hospitals have compromised patient care in their attempts to improve productivity.

In line with this trend, BIDMC netted millions in short-term financial improvements with implementation of the Genesis plan. With regard to its labor costs in particular, it reduced its budget by 3.35 million dollars in fiscal year 1999. But at what long-term cost?

With these changes, the hospital alienated a significant number of its nurses. With less and less organizational support, delivering the care that met their personal and professional standards exacted a huge personal cost to registered nurses, who were already shouldering an escalating burden of care. At BIDMC, nurses' typical workdays were rushed, frenzied, and exhausting.

Dissatisfaction and burnout drove many of the more experienced nurses in this study to reduce their hours, making their jobs part-time or per diem (on call). Nurses sacrificed the benefits associated with full-time work to have more control over their schedules and to reduce their exposure to the aggravating work conditions and the fast pace. The decreasing involvement of these highly qualified nurses in the nursing workforce is problematic, given the decision by many of their colleagues to leave the profession altogether and the scarcity of new nurses in the pipeline.

BIDMC had hoped to see cost savings from labor reductions. While the hospital achieved that goal in the short term, it is unclear that they will benefit from these cuts in the long term. Recruiting nurses has become a more expensive proposition as the competition to attract a dwindling population of professionals becomes fiercer. Signing bonuses, higher salaries, and the costs of advertising alone may eventually undo the hospital's financial gains as it tries to fill the vacant jobs—jobs nurses no longer seem to want.

Nor is money the only concern. Conditions that increase the already heavy demands on nurses, reduce their control over their work, and strip them of the emotional rewards of connecting to and caring for patients pose challenges to professional nursing practice. These conditions limit the ability of the skilled and competent nurses already working in hospitals to exercise their professional judgment and provide the care they deem necessary. Moreover, these conditions threaten to drive these skilled, committed people away from the bedside. Ironically, these same negative conditions demand greater reliance on nurses' commitment and professionalism: Nurses' commitment to patients and high professional standards compel them to stay late or work faster and harder to compensate for the deficiencies in hospital systems that restrict the care that patients receive.

It is unlikely that unlicensed assistants, with a minimum of training and no professional socialization, would have either the commitment or the knowledge required to overcome the same sets of problems and provide the same level of care. And what about new recruits to nursing?

Throwing money at the problem of recruiting and retaining nurses will not provide a meaningful solution unless the underlying issues in nurses' work are addressed. Who will be attracted to nursing if the profession is stripped of its most attractive features? Will they enter the field with the same level of professionalism and commitment to patients if they know they are entering a job that, at best, makes it difficult to act upon these motivations? And what type of care will nurses give patients if their chief incentive for entering the field is money?

These same questions pertain to the futures of other caring professions employed by resource-strapped organizations that have tried to change the way work is done. To the extent that these organizations try to wring productivity out of these professionals while exploiting their commitment and professionalism to maintain quality, these other caring professions, such as teaching, social work, and medicine—will (or have already) also become less attractive, less able to retain and attract the best and brightest. While employing organizations claim they cannot afford the time-intensive caring that these professionals value, the question is whether our society can afford to continue the cost-saving practices that strip these aspects from professionals' work and deny them to the vulnerable and needy populations that these professionals want so badly to serve.

BIDMC may be in better shape than many hospitals going through similar changes due to the high level of education and experience of its nursing staff. Approximately 73 percent of the nursing staff at BIDMC have attained a Bachelor's of Science in Nursing or higher level of education, compared to a national average of 34 percent for all hospitals and 59 percent for magnet hospitals (Bednash 2000). The high level of professionalism, knowledge, and skill of the nurses at BIDMC may help them compensate for the problems they are encountering in the hospital system more easily than a novice or less-educated staff. But how long will this last? How long will veteran nurses stay at the hospital? How will new recruits fare if they do not have educated, experienced nurses to guide them?

It seems that BIDMC leadership may, in the end, have realized some of the errors in their approach to organizational restructuring. In March 2001, Reinertsen, then CEO of CareGroup and of BIDMC, did something remarkable. He wrote an op-ed piece for the *Boston Globe* about the impending nursing shortage and the vital importance of nurses and their relationships with patients:

> In order for our patients to be safe, to attain the best possible outcomes, and to feel cared for, [hospitals] must be well-staffed by highly trained, technically skilled, compassionate nurses. And nurses, in turn, need an environment that recognizes their extraordinary responsibility for patient safety and contribution to the healing process, an environment that accords them full membership on the team of health care professionals.[7]

[7] James L. Reinertsen, "A Looming Nursing Crisis," *Boston Globe,* 15 March 2001, A19.

In Reinertsen's discussion of the looming nursing shortage, do we detect a sort of apology to BIDMC's nurses? Perhaps a recognition of the mistake BIDMC made in dismantling the Nursing Department and trying to squeeze production-line–type efficiency out of its nurses? In his article, Reinertsen validates the claims that BIDMC nurses made during my fieldwork that in order to provide excellent care to patients—care that promoted comfort and recovery—nurses needed influence, resources, and respect for their professional judgment and level of responsibility.

Reinertsen recognizes "a central lesson in health care—that effective health care depends on the development of healing relationships, one by one, between health professionals and those who come to us for care."[8] This emphasis on healing relationships contrasts with administrators' claims, during the time of my fieldwork, that nurses could not and did not need to spend significant amounts of time at the bedside developing relationships with patients and their families. Reinertsen goes a step further in emphasizing the importance of nurses' relationships with patients: "And in those instances when we cannot cure, nurses' relationships with patients and families help us to make sure we can heal."[9] Rabkin and Clifford would have been proud. Except that this recognition was too little and came far too late.

Reinertsen tells us that hospitals "with a historic tradition of nursing excellence can provide us with a blueprint for action" for attracting and retaining nurses. This insight came, however, only after BIDMC had deconstructed the nursing structure that supported nursing excellence. It came after BIDMC pushed out all of the architects of Beth Israel's successful blueprint for action for retaining and attracting nurses. Clifford had moved on from her post at CareGroup to start the Institute for Nursing Healthcare Leadership. Gibbons, her successor at BIDMC, had been fired in September 2000 and had been quickly snapped up by Massachusetts General Hospital—one of BIDMC's fiercest competitors—where she was later joined by many of Beth Israel's most seasoned nurse administrators. Finally, this insight came just as Reinertsen would lose his ability to act on it. His article was published a mere four months before he himself was fired.

[8] Ibid.
[9] Ibid.

If there is good news for nurses in all of this, it is that Paul Levy, the new chief executive of BIDMC as of January 2002, also seems to know the value of his nurses. The Hunter Group—a consulting firm famous (or, depending upon one's perspective, infamous) for designing dramatic turnaround plans for organizations on their deathbeds—spent three months in 2002 evaluating BIDMC's situation and outlining a plan for the hospital to close its budget gap, which threatens to top $146 million by 2004. They judged that if BIDMC could not right itself in six months, it should be sold to a for-profit hospital chain. Levy deemed some of the Hunter Group's recommendations unnecessary and unrealistic. One of the recommendations he rejected was laying off 15 percent of the nursing staff, 150 nurses. Levy said that such cuts would endanger patients.[10]

There are hopeful signs that BIDMC will recover from its state of financial emergency.[11] And, as the hospital shows some signs of economic recovery, it is also publicly emphasizing its esteem for its nurses. In September and October 2002, BIDMC, as a sponsor of the local National Public Radio station, aired a promotion "saluting its nurses and caregivers for their extraordinary dedication and commitment to patient care." If there is action behind these sentiments, then perhaps BIDMC can reclaim a reputation in the eyes of nurses, caregivers, and patients as a caring and competent institution.

Dianne Anderson, who accepted the role of nurse executive and Vice President of Patient Care Services at BIDMC in May 2001, reports that "nursing is a major organizational focus" at the hospital right now and that BIDMC is striving to become "the employer of choice" for nurses (personal communication, October 11, 2002). Even if BIDMC succeeds in once again building an exemplary nursing program—one that maximizes nurses' satisfaction and patients' comfort and safety while also meeting cost constraints—larger issues remain.

Forced to compete to fill vacant nursing positions, many hospitals may develop interest in becoming employers of choice in their markets. In the short term, they may devote more resources to improving nurses' work conditions than they have in the past. They may even succeed in making

[10] Liz Kowalczyk, "Beth Israel Found Long on Staffing, Short on Vision," *Boston Globe,* 10 January 2002, A1.

[11] Steve Bailey, "A Hospital Heals Itself," *Boston Globe,* 6 September 2002, E1.

hospital nursing a more attractive career. What about the long term? Will hospitals still direct resources to nursing if there are enough or even a surplus of nurses to meet demand? Will nurses still wield influence over hospital policies and patient care if there is no shortage? Meaningful change requires that organizational support for nurses and their work be lasting, designed to weather changes in hospital leadership and finances.

Appendix

Studying Change at BIDMC

In June 1998, I approached the Nursing Service at BIDMC about studying the impact of the Beth Israel–Deaconness merger on the nurses there. Even two years in, the merger hung like a thundercloud over BIDMC, with worried personnel wondering when the storm would hit. Although the hospitals had merged names and administration, few changes had taken place because the leadership hoped to ease everyone comfortably into the changes. But the slow pace was causing anxiety and anger among the staff. The nursing leadership recognized the discord among the nurse managers from the two hospitals and the sinking morale among the rank and file, but they did not have the time or resources to investigate the problem. They welcomed and encouraged my interest, hoping my results would help identify problems and point to solutions.

Although I had initially intended to study the effects of the merger on nurses, the hospital faced other monumental changes that also might affect frontline nurses. Studying a changing organization is much like trying to paint a still life in the midst of an earthquake. There was a lot happening at BIDMC and at a rapid pace. Understanding the consequences of hospital restructuring for nurses required a careful examination of what had changed and what these changes meant. I spent nine months, from January through September 1999, collecting data at BIDMC.

Open-ended interviews with seventy-seven employees at BIDMC provide the core data for this research. Because I expected that individuals' responses to organizational restructuring would be shaped in part by structural features of their position in the organization, I selected individuals situated in different positions in the organizational hierarchy. In order to get a balanced view of the impact of the merger and consequent restructuring, I spoke with an almost equal number of people from each premerger hospital, thirty-six from the former Beth Israel Hospital and thirty-four from the former New England Deaconess Hospital. All interviewees were guaranteed anonymity (pseudonyms are used for interviewee names), and only four of the individuals approached for interviews declined.

Because I expected that individuals occupying different positions in the hospital hierarchy might have distinct perspectives on changes, I interviewed thirty-four nurses, sixteen administrators (eight from the nursing service), ten nurse managers, and seventeen other members of the health care team (e.g., physicians, social workers, case managers, and patient care coworkers). Since most of the current leadership was from the former Beth Israel hospital or was new to the scene, I interviewed several additional nurse managers and nursing leaders from the former New England Deaconess Hospital, many of whom had left their previous positions. However, my focus on the survivors of organizational change dictated that most interviews were with current employees of BIDMC. This interview sampling strategy helped me develop a more rounded view of the merger dynamics and cultural differences between the two hospitals.

Different units within the hospital were exposed to restructuring to different extents, which could create differences in nurses' experiences on those units. To explore this potential range of experiences, I used an embedded case study design (Yin 1994) of six units at BIDMC. Although the units had different practice areas, all served the adult, inpatient medical surgical population. This similarity in patient population facilitated comparing organizational arrangements and work conditions across the units. When my fieldwork began in January 1999, the units involved in this study accounted for one-third of the inpatient units in the hospital. These six units represented over one-fourth of the nursing staff working with the inpatient adult population, and just under one-fifth of the nursing staff in the entire hospital.

By the end of my fieldwork, only three inpatient units at BIDMC had consolidated with their counterparts from the other premerger hospital. Two of these units—the Emergency Department, which consolidated in

1997, and the Cardiothoracic Unit, which consolidated in 1999 while I was conducting fieldwork—are included in the sample of units studied. The remaining four units included Neuromedicine, Neurosurgery, General Medicine, and Vascular Surgery (including the Vascular Intensive Care Unit).[1]

In addition to collecting data from a variety of informants, I also used multiple methods to allow for data triangulation, "the checking of inferences drawn from one set of data sources by collecting data from others" (Hammersley and Atkinson 1995:230). Each of the research methods approached the question of changes and their effects from a different angle, thereby widening the research perspective and limiting the potential of any one line of questioning or source bias to exercise too great an influence on results. I conducted participant observation, interviews, focus groups, and surveys on each of the six units in the sample, and I also used a variety of internal hospital data sources.

Through observation, I examined differences in the way the units operated, in procedures and behaviors among nurses, and in work pace and stress. During observations, I shadowed individual nurses as they went about their daily routines and observed their work processes and interactions with patients and other members of the care team. While I mostly observed nurses on the day shift, I also tailed nurses during the evening and night shifts. Following nurses on different shifts allowed me to examine potential differences in work conditions and unit operation at those times.

On each of the units, I interviewed at least three nurses, the nurse manager, and at least one other staff member on the unit (e.g., a case manager, nursing assistant, or a physician). This sampling strategy allowed me to get the perspectives of the staff nurses and the people who supervised and worked with them on a daily basis. Encounters during my observations and recommendations of nurse managers and staff helped identify individuals with knowledge or experience relevant to my research questions and guided my selection of individuals for interviews. For the majority of interviews with nurses, I selected experienced nurses who had been at the

[1] Technically, this is two units, but the vascular Intensive Care Unit is in close proximity to the vascular surgery unit and shares the same nurse manager and some of the same staff. Therefore, I analyze these two units as one setting and refer to them as one unit.

hospital since before the merger. I also made a point of interviewing several more recently hired nurses to compare their views about the quality of care and the situation at the hospital.

Open-ended interview questions provided information on what informants believed had changed at the hospital since the merger. I asked the same basic set of questions of all informants. (See Weinberg 2000 for all research protocols used in this study). However, the typical interview involved numerous interruptions; for example, pagers going off, phone calls, patients' families requesting information, patient care coworkers requiring assistance. Therefore, interviews needed to be as flexible as possible to respect people's work obligations. Interviews probed what had changed at the hospital, on the unit, and in particular for each informant. The protocol also focused attention on the relationships among coworkers and on the status and autonomy of nurses.

Often, before an interview, informants warned they had very little time, but most became engrossed in the interview and stayed beyond this limit. Some interviewees became emotional during the interview; several even cried. Informants seemed invested in their accounts of events at the hospital. Some informants may have used interviews as a forum to gripe, whereas others may have downplayed problems. While, no doubt, some of both scenarios occurred, participant observation provided balance (Hammersley and Atkinson 1995). I often incorporated events I observed into interview questions and asked informants to reconcile their accounts with those events. At the same time, interviews informed interpretation of my observations and sensitized me to things to watch.

While interviews addressed changes since the merger, focus groups concentrated on nurses' work conditions and ability to provide high-quality patient care. I conducted focus groups on each of the six units during working hours. A total of thirty-eight nurses, at least six on each unit, participated in the focus groups. These groups gathered to discuss their definitions of good nursing care, the factors necessary to facilitate it, and the extent to which good care was provided on their units.

The group dynamics in focus groups differentiated them from individual interviews. Nurses bounced ideas off each other during these group discussions, often finishing each other's thoughts or being reminded of events that had occurred. While private interviews might encourage exaggeration of problems, speaking before a group of peers might encourage minimization of experiences with quality-of-care problems.

Surveys expanded the reach of this research to the larger sample of nurses working on the six study units, not just the ones that I could interview individually or who could attend focus groups. The survey was based largely on the Outcomes of Hospital Care, Staff Registered Nurse Questionnaire used by Linda Aiken and her colleagues at the Center for Health Services and Policy Research at the University of Pennsylvania (see, e.g., Aiken, Sochalski, and Lake 1997). Their survey includes a slightly modified form of the Nursing Work Index (NWI) developed by Marlene Kramer and Laurin Hafner (1989) in their study of magnet hospitals. The NWI had been administered at Beth Israel Hospital in 1986, and within the University of Pennsylvania survey, in 1991 and 1998. Drs. Aiken and Sochalski of the University of Pennsylvania provided me with the survey data from 1986 and 1991, thereby allowing for an examination of changes in organizational arrangements over time (see Table 1 in Chapter 8).

I administered closed-ended surveys on the six study units to all of the staff registered nurses identified by the nurse manager as working regularly on the unit, for a total of 217 surveys. Surveys were anonymous, as requested by the Nursing Research Review Committee. Some 147 surveys were returned, for a total response rate of 67.5 percent. The anonymity of the surveys may have supported more candid responses than face-to-face encounters.

I used the surveys to assess the pervasiveness of the perspectives and experiences expressed in interviews and focus groups and witnessed during my observations. Many of the survey questions complement questions from the interviews and focus groups. The survey results speak to the perceptions in 1999 of a larger group of nurses about current organizational arrangements and their effects.

Finally, I used BIDMC newsletters, bulletins, internal memos, meeting minutes, and nursing division records to document actual changes, not just participants' perceptions of changes, at the hospital. These archival data lend some historical perspective to the analysis and could be used to reflect the accuracy of my informants' and my own observations.

References

Abbott, Andrew. 1988. The *System of Professions: An Essay on the Division of Expert Labor.* Chicago: University of Chicago Press.

Ad Hoc Committee to Defend Health Care. 1997. "Policy Perspectives: For Our Patients, Not for Profits: A Call to Action." *Journal of the American Medical Association* 278:1733–1738.

Aiken, Linda, Sean P. Clarke, Douglas M. Sloane, Julie A. Sochalski, Reinhard Busse, Heather Clarke, Phyllis Giovanetti, Jennifer Hunt, Anne Marie Rafferty, and Judith Shamian. 2001. "Nurses' Reports on Hospital Care in Five Countries." *Health Affairs* 20(3):43–53.

Aiken, Linda, and Claire M. Fagin. 1997. "Evaluating the Consequences of Hospital Restructuring." *Medical Care* 35:OS1–OS4.

Aiken, Linda H., Eileen T. Lake, Julie Sochalski, and Douglas M. Sloane. 1997. "Design of an Outcomes Study of the Organization of Hospital AIDS Care." *Research in the Sociology of Health Care* 14:3–26.

Aiken, Linda H., and Douglas M. Sloane. 1997a. "Effects of Organizational Innovations in AIDS Care on Burnout Among Urban Hospital Nurses." *Work and Occupations* 24:453–477.

——. 1997b. "Effects of Specialization and Client Differentiation on the Status of Nurses: the Case of AIDS." *Journal of Health and Social Behavior* 38:203–222.

Aiken, Linda H., Douglas M. Sloane., and Eileen T. Lake. 1997. "Satisfaction with Inpatient Acquired Immunodeficiency Syndrome Care." *Medical Care* 35:948–962.

Aiken, Linda H., Douglas M. Sloane., Eileen T. Lake, Julie Sochalski, and Anita L. Weber. 1999. "Organization and Outcomes in Inpatient AIDS Care." *Medical Care* 37:760–772.

Aiken, Linda H., Herbert L. Smith, and Eileen T. Lake. 1994. "Lower Medicare Mortality among a Set of Hospitals Known for Good Nursing Care." *Medical Care* 32:771–787.

Aiken, Linda H., Julie Sochalski, and Gerard F. Anderson. 1996. "Downsizing the Hospital Nursing Workforce." *Health Affairs* 15(4):88–92.

Aiken, Linda H., Julie Sochalski, and Eileen T. Lake. 1997. "Studying Outcomes of Organizational Change in Health Services." *Medical Care* 35(supp.):NS6–NS18.

Alexander, Jeffrey, and Shoou-Yih D. Lee. 1996. "The Effects of CEO Succession and Tenure on Failure of Rural Community Hospitals." *Journal of Applied Behavioral Science* 32:70–88.

American Hospital Association. 1999. *Hospital Statistics*. Chicago: Health Forum.

Anspach, Renee. 1996. *Deciding Who Lives: Fateful Choices in the Intensive Care Nursery*. Berkeley: University of California Press.

Appelbaum, Eileen, and Rosemary Batt. 1994. *The New American Workplace: Transforming Work Systems in the United States*. Ithaca: ILR Press.

Barro, Jason R., and David M. Cutler. 1997. "Consolidation in the Medical Care Marketplace: A Case Study From Massachusetts." *National Bureau of Economic Research, Inc., Working Paper Series #5957*.

Bazzoli, Gloria J., Anthony LoSasso, Richard Arnould, and Madeleine Shalowitz. 2002. "Hospital Reorganization and Restructuring Achieved Through Merger." *Health Care Management Review* 27(1):7-20.

Bednash, Geraldine. 2000. "The Decreasing Supply of Registered Nurses: Inevitable Future or Call to Action?" *Journal of the American Medical Association* 283:2985–2987.

Blegen, Mary A., Colleen J. Goode, and Laura Reed. 1998. "Nurse Staffing and Patient Outcomes." *Nursing Research* 47:43–50.

Blumenthal, David, and Gregg S. Meyer. 1996. "Academic Health Centers in a Changing Environment." *Health Affairs* 15(2):200–214.

Bogue, Richard J., Stephen M. Shortell, Min-Woong Sohn, Larry M. Manheim, Gloria Bazzoli, and Cheeling Chan. 1995. "Hospital Reorganization after Merger." *Medical Care* 33:676–686.

Brannon, Robert L. 1994. *Intensifying Care: The Hospital Industry, Professionalization, and the Reorganization of the Nursing Labor Process*. Amityville, N.Y.: Baywood.

Braverman, Harry. [1974] 1998. *Labor and Monopoly Capital: The Degradation of Work in the Twentieth Century*. New York: Monthly Review Press.

Buerhaus, Peter I., and Douglas O. Staiger. 1999. "Trouble in the Nurse Labor Market? Recent Trends and Future Outlook." *Health Affairs* 18(1):214–222.

Buerhaus, Peter I., Douglas O. Staiger, and David I. Auerbach. 2000. "Implications of an Aging Registered Nurse Workforce." *Journal of the American Medical Association* 283:2948–2954.

Buono, Anthony F., and James L. Bowditch. 1989. *The Human Side of Mergers and Acquisitions: Managing Collisions Between People, Cultures, and Organizations*. San Francisco: Jossey-Bass.

Buono, Anthony F., and Aaron J. Nurick. 1992. "Intervening in the Middle: Coping Strategies in Mergers and Acquisitions." *Human Resource Planning* 15(2):19–34.

Burns, Lawton R., Gloria J. Bazzoli, Linda Dynan, and Douglas R. Wholey. 1997. "Managed Care, Market Stages, and Integrated Delivery Systems: Is There a Relationship?" *Health Affairs* 16(6):204–218.

Cartwright, Sue, and Cary L. Cooper. 1993. "The Psychological Impact of Merger and Acquisition on the Individual: A Study of Building Society Managers." *Human Relations* 46:327–348.

Chambliss, Daniel F. 1996. *Beyond Caring: Hospitals, Nurses, and the Social Organization of Ethics*. Chicago: University of Chicago Press.

Clifford, Joyce C. 1990. "Professionalizing a Nursing Service: An Integrated Approach for the Management of Patient Care." In *Advancing Professional Nursing Practice: Innovations at Boston's Beth Israel Hospital,* edited by Joyce C. Clifford and Kathy J. Horvath, 30–50. New York: Springer.

——. 1998. *Restructuring: The Impact of Hospital Organization on Nursing Leadership*. Chicago: American Hospital Publishing, Inc.

Covin, Teresa Joyce, Kevin W. Sightler, Thomas A. Kolenko, and Tudor R Keith. 1996. "An Investigation of Post-Acquisition Satisfaction With the Merger." *Journal of Applied Behavioral Science* 32:125–143.

Curtin, Leah, and Roy Simpson. 2000. "Staffing and the Quality of Care." *Health Management Technology* 21(5):42–45.

Donelan, Karen, Robert J. Blendon, George D. Lundberg, David R. Calkins, Joseph P. Newhouse, Lucian Leape, Dahlia K. Remler, and Humphrey Taylor. 1997. "The New Medical Marketplace: Physicians' Views." *Health Affairs* 16(5):139–148.

Dranove, David, Amy Durkac, and Mark Shanley. 1996. "Perspective: Are Multihospital Systems More Efficient?" *Health Affairs* 15:100–104.

Duke, Kathryn Saenz. 1996. "Snapshots: Hospitals in a Changing Health Care System." *Health Affairs* 15(2):49–61.

Fennell, Mary L., and Jeffrey A. Alexander. 1993. "Perspectives on Organizational Change in the U.S. Medical Care Sector." *Annual Review of Sociology* 19:89–112.

Freidson, Eliot. 1970. *Profession of Medicine: A Study of the Sociology of Applied Knowledge*. New York: Harper and Row.

Good, Mary-Jo Delvecchio. [1995] 1998. *American Medicine: The Quest For Competence*. Berkeley: University of California Press.

Gordon, Suzanne. 1997. *Life Support: Three Nurses on the Front Lines*. Boston: Back Bay Books.

Gray, Bradford H. 1991. *The Profit Motive and Patient Care: The Changing Accountability of Doctors and Hospitals*. Cambridge: Harvard University Press.

Greene, Jay. 1992. "The Costs of Hospital Mergers." *Modern Healthcare* 22(5):36–43.

Guterman, Stuart, Jack Ashby, and Timothy Greene. 1996. "Hospital Cost Growth Down." *Health Affairs* 15(3):134–139.

Guzzo, Richard A., Richard D. Jette, and Raymond A. Katzell. 1985. The Effects of Psychologically Based Intervention Programs on Worker Productivity: A Meta-Analysis. *Personnel Psychology* 38:275–291.

Hallam, Kristen. 1999. "Givebacks: Healthcare Wins on Medicare, Wants More." *Modern Healthcare* 29(48):3–4.

Hammersley, Martyn, and Paul Atkinson. 1995. *Ethnography: Principles in Practice*. 2d ed. New York: Routledge.

Harkness, Gail A., Judith Miller, and Nadine Hill. 1992. "Differentiated Practice: A Three-Dimensional Model." *Nursing Management* 23(12):26–27, 30.

Joint Commission on Accreditation of Healthcare Organizations. 2002. *Health Care at the Crossroads: Strategies for Addressing the Nursing Crisis*.

Kanter, Rosabeth Moss. 1977. *Men and Women of the Corporation*. New York: Basic Books.

Kanter, Rosabeth Moss, Barry A. Stein, and Todd D. Jick, eds. 1992. *The Challenge of Organizational Change: How Companies Experience It and Leaders Guide It*. New York: Free Press.

Katz, Daniel, and Robert L. Kahn. 1978. *The Social Psychology of Orgainzations*. 2d ed. Chichester, United Kingdom: John Wiley and Sons.

Kelly, John. 1992. "Does Job Re-Design Theory Explain Job Re-Design Outcomes?" *Human Relations* 45:753–773.

King, Gary, James Honaker, Anne Joseph, and Kevin Scheve. 2001. "Analyzing Incomplete Political Science Data: An Alternative Algorithm for Multiple Imputation." *American Political Science Review* 95:49–69.

Kohn, Linda T., Janet M. Corrigan, and Molla S. Donaldson, eds. 2000. *To Err Is Human: Building a Safer Health System*. Washington, D.C.: Institute of Medicine.

Kovner, Christine, and Peter J. Gergen. 1998. "Nurse Staffing Levels and Adverse Events Following Surgery in U.S. Hospitals." *Image: Journal of Nursing Scholarship* 30:315–321.

Kramer, Marlene, and Laurin P. Hafner. 1989. "Shared Values: Impact on Staff Nurse Job Satisfaction and Perceived Productivity." *Nursing Research* 38(3):172–177.

Kramer, Marlene, and Claudia Schmalenberg. 1988. "Magnet Hospitals: Institutions of Excellence Part I." *Journal of Nursing Administration* 18(1):13–24.

Kuttner, Robert. 1999. "The American Health Care System—Wall Street and Health Care." *New England Journal of Medicine* 340:664–668.

Lee, Shoou-Yih D., and Jeffrey A. Alexander. 1999. "Managing Hospitals in Turbulent Times: Do Organizational Changes Improve Hospital Survival?" *Health Services Research* 34:923–946.

Leicht, Kevin T., Mary L. Fennell, and Kristine M. Witkowski. 1995. "The Effects of Hospital Characteristics and Radical Organizational Change on the Relative Standing of Health Care Professions." *Journal of Health and Social Behavior* 36:151–167.

Levit, Katharine, Cathy Cowan, Helen Lazenby, Arthur Sesenig, Patricia McDonnell, Jean Stiller, Anne Martin, and the Health Accounts Team. 2000. "Health Spending in 1998: Signals of Change." *Health Affairs* 19(1):124–132.

Levit, Katharine, Helen C. Lazenby, Bradley R. Braden, and the National Health Accounts Team. 1998. "National Health Spending Trends in 1996." *Health Affairs* 17(1):35–51.

Lubatkin, Michael H., and Peter J. Lane. 1996. "Psst . . . The Merger Mavens Still Have It Wrong." *Academy of Management Executive* 10:21–37.

MacDonald, Keith. 1995. *The Sociology of the Professions*. Thousand Oaks, Calif.: Sage.

Marks, Mitchell Lee, and Philip H. Mirvis. 1992. "Rebuilding after the Merger: Dealing with 'Survivor Sickness.'" *Organizational Dynamics* 21(2):18–33.

Maslach, Christina, and Susan E. Jackson. 1981. "The Measurement of Experienced Burnout." *Journal of Occupational Behaviour* 2:99–113.

Mick, Stephen S. 1990. "Themes, Issues, and Research Avenues." In *Innovations in Health Care Delivery: Insights for Organizational Theory,* edited by Stephen S. Mick and Associates, 1–19. San Francisco: Jossey-Bass.

Miller, Katherine I., and Peter R. Monge. 1986. "Participation, Satisfaction, and Productivity: A Meta-Analytic Review." *Academy of Management Journal* 29:727–753.

Needleman, Jack, Peter Buerhaus, Soeren Mattke, Maureen Stewart, and Katya Zelevinsky. 2002. "Nurse Staffing Levels and the Quality of Care in Hospitals." *New England Journal of Medicine* 346:1715–1720.

Neuman, George A., Jack E. Edwards, and Nambury S. Raju. 1989. "Organizational Development Interventions: A Meta-Analysis of Their Effects on Satisfaction and Other Attitudes. *Personnel Psychology* 42:461–489.

Norrish, Barbara R., and Thomas G. Rundall. 2001. "Hospital Restructuring and the Work of Registered Nurses." *Milbank Quarterly* 79:55–79.

Porter, Sam. 1995. *Nursing's Relationship with Medicine: A Critical Realist Ethnography.* Brookfield, Vermont: Avebury.

Primm, Peggy L. 1987. "Differentiated Practice for AND- and BSN- Prepared Nurses." *Journal of Professional Nursing* 3:218–224.

Prospective Payment Assessment Commission (PROPAC). 1997. *Medicare and the American Health Care System—Report to the Congress, June 1997.* Washington: Government Printing Office.

Rabkin, Mitchell T. 1990. "Ascent from Mediocrity: A Redefinition of Nursing." In *Advancing Professional Nursing Practice: Innovations At Boston's Beth Israel Hospital,* edited by Joyce C. Clifford and Kathy J. Horvath, 3–13. New York: Springer.

Reuter, James, and Darrell Gaskin. 1997. "Academic Health Centers in Competitive Markets." *Health Affairs* 16(4):242–252.

Robertson, Peter J., Darryl R. Roberts, and Jerry I. Porras. 1993. "Dynamics of Planned Organizational Change: Assessing Empirical Support for a Theoretical Model." *Academy of Management Journal* 36:619–634.

Robertson, Randal H., Steven B. Dowd, and Mahmud Hassan. 1997. "Skill-Specific Staffing Intensity and the Cost of Hospital Care." *Health Care Management Review* 22(4):61–71.

Robinson, James C. 1994. "The Changing Boundaries of the American Hospital." *Milbank Quarterly* 73:131–160.

Robinson, James C., and Lawrence P. Casalino. 1996. "Vertical Integration and Organizational Networks in Health Care." *Health Affairs* 15(1):7–22.

Rothman, Robert A., Allen M. Schwartzbaum, and John H. McGrath III. 1971. "Physicians and a Hospital Merger: Patterns of Resistance to Organizational Change." *Journal of Health and Social Behavior* 12:46–55.

Rubin, Donald B. 1987. *Multiple Imputation for Nonresponse in Surveys*. New York: John Wiley and Sons.

Salancik, Gerald R., and Jeffrey Pfeffer. 1977. "Who Gets Power and How They Hold on to It: A Strategic-Contingency Model of Power." *Organizational Dynamics* 6:2–21.

Schafer, J. L. 1997. *Analysis of Incomplete Multivariate Data*. New York: Chapman and Hall.

——. 1999. NORM: Multiple imputation of incomplete multivariate data under a normal model, version 2. Software for Windows 95/98/NT, available from http://www.stat.psu.edu/~jls/misoftwa.html.

Scott, Robert A., Linda H. Aiken, David Mechanic, and Julius Moravcsik. 1995. "Organizational Aspects of Caring." *Milbank Quarterly* 73:77–95.

Shindul-Rothschild, Judith, Diane Berry, and Ellen Long-Middleton. 1996. "Where Have All the Nurses Gone? Final Results of Our Patient Care Survey." *American Journal of Nursing* 96(11):25–39.

Shortell, Stephen M., Robin R. Gillies, and Kelly J. Devers. 1995. "Reinventing the American Hospital." *Milbank Quarterly* 73:131–160.

Shortell, Stephen M., Robin R. Gillies, David A. Anderson, Karen Morgan Erickson, and John B. Mitchell. 1997. *Remaking Health Care in America: Building Organized Delivery Systems*. San Francisco: Jossey-Bass.

Sochalski, Julie, Linda H. Aiken, and Claire M. Fagin. 1997. "Hospital Restructuring in the United States, Canada, and Western Europe." *Medical Care* 35:OS13–OS25.

Spang, Heather Radach, Gloria J. Bazzoli, and Richard J. Arnould. 2001. "Hospital Mergers and Savings for Consumers: Exploring New Evidence." *Health Affairs* 20(4):150–159.

Spector, Paul E. 1986. "Perceived Control By Employees: A Meta-Analysis of

Studies Concerning Autonomy and Participation at Work." *Human Relations* 39:1005–1016.

Starr, Paul. 1982. *The Social Transformation of American Medicine: The Rise of a Sovereign Profession and the Making of a Vast Industry.* New York: Basic Books.

Stone, Deborah. 1999. "Care and Trembling." *The American Prospect* 43 (March-April):61–67.

Tarnow-Mordi; W. O, C. Hau; A. Warden; A. J. Shearer. 2000. "Hospital Mortality in Relation to Staff Workload: A 4-Year Study in an Adult Intensive-Care Unit." *Lancet* 35: 185–189.

Topping, Sharon, and S. Robert Hernandez. 1991. "Health Care Strategy Research, 1985–1990: A Critical Review." *Medical Care Review* 48:47–89.

Wagner, John A. III. 1994. "Participation's Effects on Performance and Satisfaction: A Reconsideration of Research Evidence." *Academy of Management Review* 19:312–330.

Wagner, John A. III, and Richard Z. Gooding. 1987. "Shared Influence and Organizational Behavior: A Meta-Analysis of Situational Variables Expected to Moderate Participation-Outcome Relationships." *Academy of Management Journal* 30:524–541.

Weinberg, Dana Beth. 2000. *Why Are the Nurses Crying? Restructuring, Power, and Control in an American Hospital.* Cambridge, Mass.: Harvard University, unpublished doctoral dissertation.

White, Kerr L. 1997. "Hospital Restructuring in North America." *Medical Care* 35:OS7–OS12.

Wicks, Deidre. 1998. *Nurses and Doctors at Work: Rethinking Professional Boundaries.* Buckingham, United Kingdom: Open University Press.

Wiggins, Marjorie Splaine, Judith M. Farias, and Judith R. Miller. 1990. "The Role of the Patient Care Technician at the New England Deaconess Hospital." In *Patient Care Delivery Models,* edited by Gloria Gilbert Mayer, Mary Jane Madden, and Eunice Lawrenz, 185–200. Rockville, Md.: Aspen.

Witz, Anne. 1992. *Professions and Patriarchy.* New York: Routledge.

Wright, John W., and Linda Sunshine. 1995. *The Best Hospitals in America: The Top-Rated Medical Facilities in the U.S. and Canada.* 2d ed. Detroit: Gale Research, Inc.

Wunderlich, Gooloo S., Frank A. Sloan, and Carolyne K. Davis, eds. 1996. *The Adequacy of Nurse Staffing in Hospitals and Nursing Homes.* Washington, D.C.: Institute of Medicine.

Yin, Robert K. 1994. *Case Study Research: Design and Methods.* 2d ed. Thousand Oaks, Calif.: Sage.

Index